The
Little Book
of Skin Care

The Little Book of Skin Care

Korean Beauty Secrets for Healthy, Glowing Skin

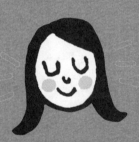

Charlotte Cho

WILLIAM MORROW
An Imprint of HarperCollinsPublishers

This book is written as a source of information only. The information contained in this book should by no means be considered a substitute for the advice of a qualified medical professional, who should always be consulted before beginning any new diet, exercise, or other health program. All efforts have been made to ensure the accuracy of the information contained in this book as of the date published. The author and the publisher expressly disclaim responsibility for any adverse effects arising from the use or application of the information contained herein.

FIRST EDITION

Designed by Leah Carlson-Stanisic

Illustrations by Gemma Correll

Library of Congress Cataloging-in-Publication Data has been applied for.

ISBN 978-0-06-241638-4

16 17 18 19   OV/RRD   10 9 8 7 6 5

To Umma and Appa,

who gave me Korea and America

and the best of both worlds

Contents

Introduction

I thought *I* was beauty obsessed, and then I experienced Seoul.

Seoul breathes beauty, and its air is skin care. In Korea, it seems that everywhere you look, multitudes of products sell the promise of flawless, dewy skin, and you only have to glance at the porcelain faces passing by on the sidewalks to know that this isn't false advertising.

A California native, I was just out of college when I moved halfway around the world to live in South Korea, and as soon as I arrived, I experienced skin culture shock. Western cultures tend to think skin care is about as much fun as flossing your teeth: just another end-of-the-day chore to rush through before bed. But in Korea, taking good care of your skin is something to be enjoyed; it isn't just beauty or vanity, but an investment in your well-being. I soon came to understand that I was now living in a country where skin care was not just about the products on your bathroom shelf, but a mindset that permeates your lifestyle, from the food you eat to the clothes you wear.

My own journey to understand Korean skin care made me a believer, and when I left Seoul, I took with me a passion to share what I had learned. This led me to start my own Korean lifestyle and beauty website and e-shop, Soko Glam, and to pursue my esthetician's license in New York. Through Soko Glam, I've been able to hear personal stories from women (and men) of all ages and all cultures who decided to follow the Korean skin-care routine and have seen their skin—and confidence—change for the better.

In the United States, when we think of skin we think of problems. When a pimple rears its ugly head right before an important date, or the first time we notice fine lines appearing, we experience panic, worry, and regret. We "fight" acne, "combat" wrinkles, and "banish" blackheads. It's us against our skin, and our only ally is an unrealistic jar of miracle cream that almost always lets us down.

Our brains are filled with marketing mumbo jumbo that's a potent combo of myth and misconception. It's no wonder that people still use skin products based on age and gender, or believe that drinking water will give your dry skin relief, because that's what we've been told for generations.

As I learned more about skin care through my esthetician training, and the more I talked to people who were totally confused about what to buy or how to use certain products, I knew I had to put all my skin-care secrets from Seoul into a book. Because, really, they shouldn't be secrets anymore.

Why Read a Book About Skin Care?

. . . .

In this book, I'll share with you how a California girl like myself became immersed in Korea's beauty culture and changed the way I saw and took care of my skin. Whether you're reading this to start your first skin-care regimen, improve the one you have, or simply learn about how another culture approaches beauty, this book will do all that and more.

Sadly, reading this book alone is not enough to improve your skin, but take heart—it's the first step. It'll take a bit of work on your part, but I'll hold your well-moisturized hand along the way. I'll guide you step-by-step through some of my best-kept Korean skin-care secrets, from night and day skin-care routines, to why your entire body, not just your face, needs exfoliation, to how to choose and then use the right moisturizer. I'll also show you how to pull off the "no-makeup makeup" look that I've seen on women in the streets of Seoul (and regularly on New York and Paris runways). I'll pair my technical esthetician knowledge with advice from Seoul beauty experts to answer your toughest questions about skin and to help provide solutions to common skin issues. Learning about Korean skin care will change the way you think about your skin and how you treat it. You'll be excited to start a routine, and once you get going, you won't want to neglect it.

If you're a little doubtful, let me assure you: Yes, you can be excited about skin. It's *only* the largest organ of your body. You ready?

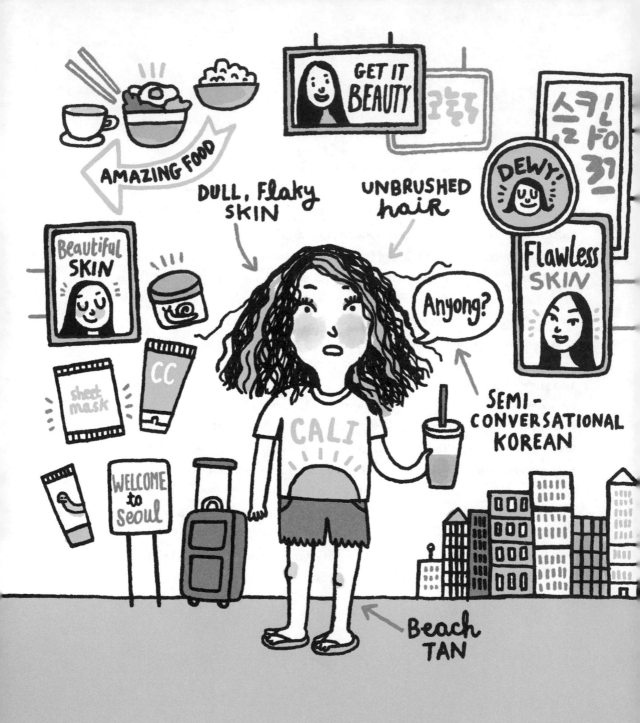

1

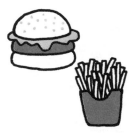

About Me:

Korean Face, California Attitude

For the first twenty-one years of my life, I was the quintessential L.A. girl. I had a year-round tan and blond highlights and lived in flip-flops. I wore cutoff shorts from Abercrombie & Fitch and sipped on vanilla milkshakes with my burger and fries, and naturally, I worshipped the beach. As soon as I could drive, I was cruising my parents' sedan to the mall, where I went shopping with the extra cash I made working as a cashier at a sushi restaurant.

When it came to beauty, I was self-taught, influenced by magazines and what I saw on the people around me. In high school, I cut asymmetrical layers in my hair and leaned over the bathroom sink to paint on chunky blond streaks with boxed drugstore dye kits. At one point, I may or may not have had a bad perm (I definitely had a perm, though how bad it was depended on whom you asked). When it came to makeup, I was definitely not going for the natural look. Instead, I opted for exaggerated heavy black eyeliner and overly tweezed eyebrows in an attempt to get that thin, Angelina Jolie–esque arch.

With my part-time job, I had the luxury to splurge on what I considered my beauty essentials: eye shadow palettes, liquid liners, juicy lip glosses, and bronzer to make my sun-kissed glow shimmer. My mom nagged me to put on sunscreen, but alas, I didn't listen. Tan was in, so instead of SPF, I'd slather on coconut-scented accelerator to make sure I got the most out of all the hours I spent at the beach.

Spaghetti with a Side of Kimchi

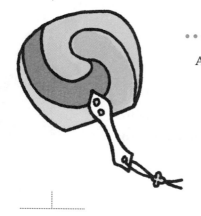

As a second-generation Korean kid (born and raised in California by Korean parents), I grew up straddling both worlds. Spaghetti nights had kimchi on the side. We celebrated New Year's on January 1 and then again for Lunar New Year. I spoke English at school but Korean at home. During my weekly ballet class, I wore the classic pink tutu, but come Saturday at Korean school, I ran around in circles waving colorful traditional *buchae*s with all the other second-gen kids who were just like me.

On occasion, and usually on Saturdays after Korean school, my mom would drag me to the local Korean-style spa, where we stood around naked with a bunch of strangers. My older sister, Michelle, relished the whole bathhouse experience, but I was not having it. The communal nudity just made me self-conscious—my barely there boobs were just starting to blossom, so the last thing I wanted to do was put them on display for the world to see.

My mom frequently lectured Michelle and me about the importance of staying out of the sun, moisturizing, and properly cleansing our faces. My older sister was much more into Korean culture than I was (she loved her Kpop boy bands) and followed dutifully, but as the middle child, I went to great lengths to do the opposite. I was determined to blaze my own trail, and going to sleep without moisturizing my face—or even (gasp!) washing it—was my forte.

My no-care skin-care regimen wasn't worth much—no surprise there—and I was a sophomore in high school when I started to get acne. There's a Korean saying that an onset of acne is a clear indication that someone has a crush, so when my dad would see my pimple-populated forehead, he would tease, "So . . . what boy were you thinking of today?"

I did have a boyfriend (shh!), so I became superstitious that my face was betraying me in some way and decided it was time to invest in some "skin care." At the local drugstore, I grabbed a bottle of the bright orange acne wash that all my friends used. We knew it was good stuff because it left your skin so tight and dry that smiling was almost painful. After a few weeks, when things weren't improving, I bought Oxy Pads, which left behind a strong burning sensation when you swiped them across your skin. As my friends said: If it stung, it was clearly working.

Needless to say, my segue into skin care abruptly stalled here. It was more trouble than it was worth, and if I had to sting and burn to fight my acne into submission, I was willing to declare defeat. Skin care was just too complicated—no one I knew seemed to know anything about it, nor did they really care to find out. My mother possessed near-perfect skin even in middle age, but I didn't think to ask her because, as all teenage girls know, moms don't know anything!

Laziness also played a huge factor in my nonchalance. Why would I obsess over perfecting my skin if I could just use concealer, foundation, and a compact for a quick fix? It was far easier to spackle makeup over my blemishes than it was to make them go away. I also had the mentality that skin care was for old people, and I still had decades before I had to worry about wrinkles.

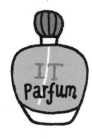

With time on my side, I put my money toward the latest "it" perfume instead, and all my friends were on the same page. With all the lip gloss and fragrance we were buying, skin care simply didn't fit into our budget, but man, did we smell good.

My skin-care game improved when I went away to college, but it turned out that it only lasted for a hot second. I was making tips as a waitress at an upscale restaurant and decided to use my newfound cash flow to dabble in expensive skin-care products. But I wasn't any less lazy; it was just that Bloomingdale's was right next door and I had money to blow. I was over-whelmed with the choices at the cosmetics counter, while a well-meaning saleswoman with her own skin issues admitted that she didn't really know what to recommend to me either. Most of her customers were women in their thirties and forties who suddenly wanted a miracle cream to get rid of crow's-feet or lift up what gravity had brought down. But I was only twenty-two, with just the vague idea that I should be taking better care of my skin. I finally walked out with an eighty-dollar bottle of toner, because my "common sense" told me that at that price, it just had to be good for my skin, even if I didn't know exactly what it was for.

With my new toner and moisturizer, and the occasional splurge (facials at a hotel spa), I felt as if I really knew how to take care of my skin, especially when I compared myself with other girls my age, who were spending their time in makeup aisles picking up the latest mascara or focusing on how their butts looked in the latest brand of designer jeans. But really, who could blame them? Why should we worry about our skin? We didn't have a wrinkle in sight!

As much as I had made the most out of living my teenage years in California, as a young adult, my beach-and-burgers existence had lost most of its charm. College felt like an extension of high school, and I started to regret sticking around my hometown. I was bored with the perfect weather, the tract housing with the same orange-yellow paint for miles, and all the strip malls. So I put my blackhead-ridden nose to the grindstone and graduated from college in just three years. I knew I had to get the hell out of there.

Skin Culture in Seoul

● ●

After I graduated, I began working at a boutique advertising agency in Orange County, but I remained on high alert for something else. An earlier trip to Seoul, the capital of South Korea and my parents' hometown, had inspired a severe case of wanderlust, and almost as soon as I got home, I was desperate to go back. I was convinced that I could claw my way to a career in Seoul and set about networking with people who had advertising connections in Korea, because ideally I wanted to live abroad there and work on my career at the same time. On a whim, I responded to an ad in a Korean English-language news daily, and just when I had almost forgotten about it, an interview request from Samsung landed in my inbox. A few weeks later, I found myself in Samsung's Houston, Texas, headquarters in front of three company VPs who seemed to think I was perfect for the international public relations job. I remember asking them timidly if my Korean "fluency" would be an issue. To my relief, they said that Samsung was such a global company, with many bilingual colleagues, that there wouldn't be a problem. Since I would be handling all international PR projects, English would be the main language.

I honestly think I landed the job because they were impressed that I paid for college by myself and finished in three years, whereas in Korea it's the custom for parents to financially care for their children until they're married, right up to paying for the wedding. Never in a million years did I think this would lead to a job offer halfway around the world, but that's exactly what happened: They wanted me to come work in Seoul. When I realized the opportunity I was just granted with this one-way ticket, I was ecstatic. In addition to what it could mean for my career, I saw this as a chance to explore the neighborhoods my parents grew up in and to eat delicious and cheap Korean food whenever I felt like it. Aside from the anticipation of filling my stomach with bibimbap, I had no idea what I was getting myself into.

When I told my parents about my plans, it would be an understatement to say that my mom and dad were confused. They'd made a lot of sacrifices in leaving Korea, and they both spent several lonely, non-English-speaking years in the United States, all in the name of creating better opportunities for the children they didn't even have yet. And then here I was, more than three decades later, dropping everything to go back to the country they thought they'd left behind for good.

I was warned that Seoul was fast-paced and overly competitive, which did concern me—what if I couldn't fit in or didn't excel at my job? Many of my friends told me I'd be homesick and predicted that I'd have a hard time meeting people. I had an aunt, uncle, and cousins (whom I hardly knew) in Korea, and when my parents let them know I was coming, they balked, saying, "Why would she come to Korea when she's got it good in America?" But in spite of all this, I couldn't have been more excited. I was convinced that the years I'd spend in Seoul—under the flashing karaoke lights, over the smoky haze of grilled pork, and on the trails along the Han River—would be the best of my life.

As I packed for my adventure, I daydreamed about being courted by a native Korean boy who had really good hair. I was certain our relationship would be a clandestine one, since he would undoubtedly turn out to be the son of a wealthy chairman and owner of Korea's largest *chaebol* (the term for "business conglomerate"). I plotted how I would battle my evil future mother-in-law so that the love her son and I had would triumph. It would be *just* like the Korean TV dramas.

When I first stepped off the plane in Seoul into a sea of shiny, black-haired heads, I had never felt more at home. The Korea my parents had left behind was a country lifting itself out of poverty, but by the time I arrived, it was a ball of energy that had sprouted concrete jungles seemingly overnight. Seoul buzzed along, fueled by the big hopes and dreams of millions of people determined to achieve them. There were endless alleys to explore, an entire culture to digest, and a plethora of welcoming cafés where I could sit and people watch. I'd expected some of this, but soon realized that my hunger wasn't just for endless Korean BBQ, but an entirely new perspective.

Then reality hit.

While I was Korean in Orange County, I was definitely American in Seoul, and I was about to experience my first bout of culture shock. I was twenty-two years old, with a beach tan, chunky highlights, and the Korean language skills of a three-year-old. I quickly found out that my semiconversational Korean was rudimentary at best.

I remember my first day at work. It was February, the dead of winter, and after navigating through the rush hour subway commute in stockings and really pinchy heels, I was pretty lost. I finally stumbled upon the correct building and was escorted by HR to meet my boss. I sat alone in a meeting room, and a man who looked a little younger than my father walked in. His name was Mr. Hong, and the respectful way to address him was Hong Boo-Jang-Nim, which meant Senior Manager Hong. In Korean, he asked, "Do you speak Korean?" I said, "A little." Then he said to me, "Well, welcome to the *hong-bo* team." "Um," I asked meekly, "what is *hong-bo*?"

"*Hong-bo* means public relations," he explained. The department he headed up. The department I would be working in. Aw, crap. And there went my chance of making a good impression. I could tell that Mr. Hong was concerned.

It turned out that despite what my interviewers had assured me, most of the *hong-bo* team did not speak English fluently, and my new colleagues were as scared about meeting me as I was about meeting them.

In California, I'd spent so much time in the sun that most people in Seoul assumed I was Southeast Asian, and at work, I was my team's first international hire. When I arrived, I think we were all surprised by just how much I didn't fit in: They had no idea what to do with me.

But I was determined to make the most of my time in Seoul and knew that I had to adapt to the city, since it wasn't going to adapt to me. It wasn't long before I was taking all the new experiences in stride. It helped that my coworkers immediately took me under their wing: My female colleagues treated me like I was their long-lost cousin—a cousin who just happened to have been raised by wolves. (Side note: Despite this rocky start, Mr. Hong and I went on to work so well together that he became a crucial partner of Soko Glam after he retired from Samsung as a sang-moonim, aka vice president.)

The people in my office teased me because I had messy, unbrushed hair, and I was met with blank stares when I tried to explain that I'd been going for the boho, beachy waves look. They thought I was barbaric because I didn't use essence in my skin-care regimen, and laughed with me (or at me?) when I admitted that I didn't even know what it was. When they asked me if I had ever been to a bathhouse or exfoliated, I opted for the easy way out and just lied. I've been recently, I said, even though the truth was that I hadn't stepped inside a Korean spa since puberty.

In passing, my coworkers would say, and rather bluntly, "I could see your dark circles from way over there," or "What is growing out of your skin?" My favorite, because it seemed to come from a place of genuine anguish about my well-being: "*Please* brush your hair."

Asian families tend to be very blunt and won't think twice about telling you you're getting fat or that you need to get a boyfriend, so rather than being offended by it, I was used to this well-intentioned rudeness, and it got me thinking about my skin. Also, since diving right into Korean culture, I'd become addicted to the soap-operatic dramas on television, and I'll admit, I was (still am) shallow enough to be influenced by the actresses. Their faces were flawless, even when I watched them in HD!

MY TOP FIVE FAVORITE KDRAMAS

1. *My Love from Another Star*
2. *Answer Me 1997*
3. *Answer Me 1994*
4. *Full House*
5. *Coffee Prince*

As I spent more time with my coworkers outside the office, I found out many of my female colleagues looked far younger than they actually were, and even my male colleagues seemed to know more about skin care than I did. It wasn't unusual for a super manly guy to have a bottle of SPF and some hand cream at his desk, and almost everyone had their own personal humidifier to keep the cold winter air from drying out their skin. The rows of cubicles were as dewy as the rain forest room at the zoo, and so were the faces. More than just dewy—they were glowing.

Outside the office, skin-care culture was just as prevalent. Every street corner in Seoul was lined with cosmetics shops—no, really, you can stand at an intersection in Myeong-dong and see the same stores every which way you turn. On my daily walk home from work, I'd pass dozens of windows filled with creams and treatments, and entering through the doors was like walking into a candy shop of mysteries. There were remedies for everything, from treating dark circles, to reducing breakouts along the chin, to CC creams that made you look flawless and natural while protecting your skin, to little gel caps that you could smooth out over your nose to get rid of blackheads. I pored through dozens of sheet masks made with rice, royal jelly, or even fermented yeast! These at-home spa facials in a packet were less than the cost of a subway ride, and they were made even more enticing by their cute and sophisticated packaging. There were potions and ingredients I'd never heard of before, like creams infused with snail extract to help fade acne scars, or snake venom to plump and firm the skin. Everything was inexpensive, and I'd spend hours in the shops, inspired to try different formulas and test the various concoctions. Even when I had a bagful of new products in my hand, I still had a list in my head of what I wanted to try next.

About Me

With so many brands and products offered, I zoned in on trying to find the best and pestered my Korean friends about their skin-care routines and the products that achieved the best results for them. I dug for information myself, going through Korean beauty blogs and watching my new favorite program, a beauty-dedicated cable show called *Get It Beauty*, which seemed to always be on in the background wherever I was. I also had teachers and allies in the shop clerks, who, despite being younger than me (or were they?), were incredibly knowledgeable about skin-care products and techniques.

The fact that skin was a priority was apparent in many day-to-day interactions. On an elevator ride up to my apartment, I eavesdropped as an older man greeted the lady standing next to me. He said to her in Korean, "Your skin looks amazing today!"

As much as I could with my peripheral vision, I examined this so-called amazing skin, which really was dewy and bright and belonged to a woman who looked to be in her late twenties, even though she could have been decades older. Her skin was so flawless and poreless, almost perfect, and her reaction showed just how much pride she took in her complexion. Her eyes widened with pleasure and she giggled at the compliment, her hand politely covering her mouth.

There were two takeaways from observing this interaction in the elevator. First, the fact that he even noticed her skin was mind-boggling. What American man would have? Second, her reaction was pure bliss. She might as well have won the lottery.

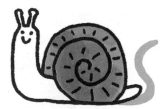

After that elevator incident, I began to notice beautiful skin everywhere I turned. So many faces I saw were silky and even. I envied how fresh and dewy they looked and wondered what these women did to keep their skin from being dull or flaky.

I know what you're thinking right now, because I thought it, too: *It's genes, dummy. They're all born with it!* But the skeptic in me was silenced every time I looked in the mirror: I was full-blooded Korean, and I was as dull and flaky as a potato. I knew I needed to start taking active steps to take care of my skin, even overhaul my regimen if needed.

Four weeks after landing in Korea, I had my own humidifier at my desk, and instead of looking forward to a glass of wine after work, I found myself genuinely excited about going home and washing my face. You know what they say: When in Seoul, do as the Koreans do.

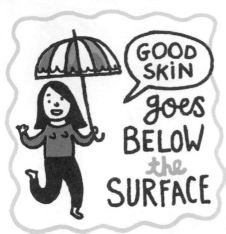

GOOD SKIN goes BELOW the SURFACE

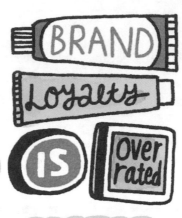

BRAND Loyalty IS over-rated

PALI Pali!

CUTE IS NOT

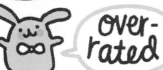

over-rated

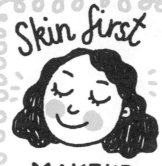

Skin first

MAKEUP second!

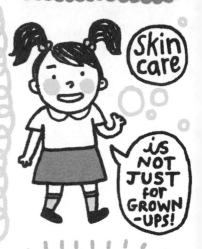

Skin care

is NOT JUST for GROWN-UPS!

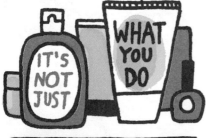

IT'S NOT JUST WHAT YOU DO

BUT HOW YOU do it

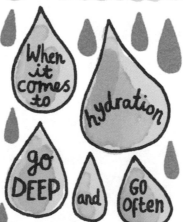

When it comes to hydration go DEEP and GO often

IT'S ABOUT BRIGHTENING

NOT Whitening

Korean Beauty 101:

The Mindset of a Skin-Obsessed Culture

*O*nce I had my feet on the ground in Seoul, it didn't take me long to realize that I was living in a place where skin care was more than skin deep: It was a part of the culture in Korea. This was a new concept, but the more I learned about it, the more excited I was to embrace it.

At the time it was the mid-2000s, and Korean beauty was just then starting to make headway in the rest of Asia, with a small yet devoted following in the United States. If you wanted Korean beauty products, you had to work for them: You could commute to stores that were overpriced and hit-or-miss, or order goods online and swallow the fact that the shipping was going to cost you more than the products themselves.

And if you didn't have a Korean friend or someone else in the know to give you insider information, well, good luck. You'd most likely be going in blind, trying to decipher labels, not knowing what the formulas were or how products were supposed to be used. You'd have to go on price alone to try to figure out which were luxury brands and which were bottom-of-the-barrel budget ones.

On my annual trips back to Los Angeles to visit my family and catch up with friends, I'd pack my suitcase full of the latest emulsions, lip tints, and eye patches. Some were long-overdue birthday gifts, but most were specific requests from friends who would sheepishly explain, "You just can't get the same stuff here for that price, so, um, can you bring me twelve?"

Other friends didn't know specifics, but had just heard that things were *c-u-t-e*. They wanted sheet masks illustrated with candy-colored snails and would text me, "I'll take anything that's shaped like a panda or a piece of fruit!!!" My arrival back in the States provoked squeals of glee from my friends, but I knew it wasn't me they were so excited about—it was that lip gloss shaped like a blueberry.

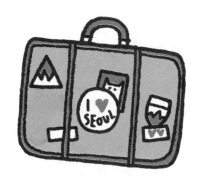

I was having the time of my life in Korea, and I had fallen in love with the country in more ways than one. It was the place where I found a husband, whom I met on a blind date. Blind dates, called *sogaeting*s, are super common in Korea. On Fridays, I'd ask my coworkers what they were up to, and often they had two or three dates lined up for a weekend. I tried my hand at a few *sogaeting*s with Korean men, but when a friend in California suggested I meet a Korean American who was a West Point graduate and captain stationed in Seoul, well, that one stuck. In

Seoul, Dave and I also found the mutual love of our life in Rambo, a poodle that we adopted from a friend.

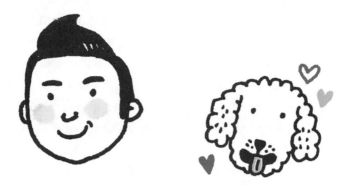

Living in Korea made me really believe in the people: I thought Korea had so much to offer the rest of the world, and I wanted to share it.

Korean skin care had become my passion. It had completely changed the way I thought about my skin and skin in general. I knew it could do the same for others, so I made it my personal mission to get that message out there. From my point of view, there was a huge gap between the United States and Korea. People were hungry for Korean products, but there was a lot of confusion and misinformation about them.

Dave and I both came from families of entrepreneurs, so we decided to take our own stab at demystifying Korean beauty: We'd open an online shop and make it easier for people in the States to find their (new) favorite products.

Rambo and I camped out on the living room floor with a pile of my all-time favorite products, the ones that I'd used for months and years, and that's where the curating started. Rambo, though he was cute, turned out to not be much of a beauty expert, so it was all on me.

At first, I thought of Soko Glam as something of a side project. My first attempts at product shots were so bad that even Dave couldn't lie and say they were good, so I found a bored owner of a small passport photo studio near my apartment and negotiated a sweet four-dollars-per-photo deal.

I wrote the product descriptions in the first person and talked about why I liked them so much and the results that I'd seen when I used them. Then I uploaded the photo studio's images and clicked publish. With that, Soko Glam was officially open for business.

The first order was from my friend Jackie and then my sister. Somehow, word spread, and when we were the focus of a small online article, orders started pouring in—from strangers! And they weren't all Korean Americans. All of a sudden, the small inventory of products that I'd stocked on the top shelf of my closet sold out completely. Whoa. It was clear that people from all backgrounds wanted Korean beauty. And they wanted it now.

In the time since we launched Soko Glam, Korean beauty had made a huge splash in the United States. *Hallyu,* which translates as "Korean Wave," refers to pop culture—from music to soap-operatic dramas, YouTube videos, and even food—that's hugely popular outside of Korea. Beauty products rode this wave like there was no tomorrow.

Korean beauty was everywhere you looked it seemed—from clickbait articles about the weirdest Korean beauty products (donkey milk for dry skin! temple viper venom for wrinkles!) to beauty blogs touting the now-famous ten-step routine (don't worry, I'll get to that in chapter seven, promise). As a result, Korean products were no longer niche. The rise in press stoked the general public's interest, and my customers were sending me lots of feedback, from e-mails to tweets to comments, about how much they loved the products they were buying.

I also realized that something unexpected but wonderful was happening: Our customers saw Soko Glam not just as a place to buy products, but to learn about skin care. They had tons of respect for Korean beauty culture and wanted to learn about their skin from that perspective.

Good Skin Goes Beyond the Surface

Korean beauty is more than just ten steps and sheet masks—it's not just what you use, but how you think. From all my experience, this is what I've come to observe about Korean beauty and the mindset that drives it. The way your skin feels and looks is priority number one. But in Korea, skin culture goes beyond products, and both men and women will go to great lengths to protect and nurture their skin. Whether they use sun umbrellas to shield themselves from UVA rays or drink antioxidant tea to prevent premature aging (and they probably do both), Koreans recognize that skin care is a holistic practice. There are several individual steps that contribute to the overall goal of beautiful skin.

Brand Loyalty Is Overrated

Korean consumers rarely stick with one brand, which keeps beauty companies on their toes. Shoppers are constantly in the market for the next best thing, and the Korean beauty industry has to develop products quickly to satisfy those needs. This also means the products have to deliver, because no one's sticking around if they don't work.

Customers also don't automatically think Korean products are superior to all other brands. There are plenty of natives who use luxury-brand cosmetics from the United States, Europe, and elsewhere. Scope out a Korean's bathroom counter or makeup bag, and you're likely to find a healthy and diverse mix of brands from home and abroad.

Pali Pali! Or, Innovation Is Everything

Korean companies can conceive a product and have it on the shelves within six months. They take full advantage of rapidly evolving technology and try to stay one step ahead of what consumers are going to want. It's all about who can be the quickest to bring a new product to market.

This means you're not going to get a plethora of products that have been around since your grandma was a girl, and there's more emphasis on new than on classic, but this is a huge part of why Korean cosmetics are so fun. You probably don't want to wear the same clothes for your entire life, so why would you want to use the same moisturizer?

Cute Is Not Overrated

Korean companies understand that packaging is important. We may be cautioned to not judge a book by its cover, but in this book, it's totally okay to judge a cheek stain by its cat ears or a mascara by its dinosaur drawings.

I'm exaggerating a bit here, because you obviously wouldn't use either of these if they were crap. But if they're good quality, why shouldn't they be cute, too? Well-designed products are more fun, and they reinforce the idea that skin care isn't just a chore, but something to be enjoyed. From hand creams to oil-blotting sheets, you carry beauty products everywhere and use them often. If you're going to have to look at something several times a day, it might as well make you smile—and if it makes you smile, you're more likely to use it. The more likely you are to use it, the more you'll see results. See? It's all part of a plot to get you healthy, glowing skin!

Skin First, Makeup Second

Instead of trying to cover up flaws with makeup and spot solutions, Koreans tend to focus on skin-care products that get at the root of conditions and treat problems before they start. Relying wholly on makeup not only looks unnatural, but it's also a temporary fix to a long-lasting issue.

This mentality is exactly why Seoul street style is filled with women who expertly pull off the "no makeup makeup" look. With their skin-care game down pat, and their basic canvas prepped and primed, they can go outside with very minimal makeup and still look flawless.

Skin Care Is Not Just for Grown-Ups

When we're kids, we're taught proper hygiene, from brushing our teeth before we go to bed to washing our hands after using the bathroom. In Korea, kids are taught about skin care as well. Long before they even have to think about adolescent acne, they're taught about everything from exfoliating and moisturizing to a generous application of SPF.

There's a pretty big difference between this and what most Western cultures consider skin care. Prevention is way more effective than treatment. Most Koreans are using SPF way before age spots start to show up and are moisturizing long before they ever have to worry about wrinkles. They're taught that, with some time and effort, you can be in control of your skin, instead of just sitting around and waiting for the day that it decides to sabotage you.

Sadly, we don't start taking care of our skin until pimples rear their heads right before prom, and then, at the first signs of aging, it's a mad dash to the store to buy the most expensive cream available. When you're young and healthy, that's when it's easiest and most beneficial to keep your body in a continuous healthy state, and your skin is no different. You know what they say: You can't teach an old dog new tricks—and the same seems to apply to skin care. If you start good habits now, they'll be second nature. Wait until you're older, and you'll be kicking and screaming your way into a skin-care routine.

It's Not Just What You Do, but How You Do It

While most people will put on a moisturizer and call it a day, Korean women use anywhere from six to ten products in their daily skin-care routine. And again, they're not just reaching for whatever's closest and slapping it on—the order in which the products are used is important, too!

From the lightest consistency to the heaviest, there's a time and place for each layer of product. Every step has a distinct purpose: prep, renew, treat, hydrate, or protect. It's also important how you apply different products—tap in your essence, pat on your eye cream, dab on your cushion compact—because slathering isn't always the best approach (we'll discuss these in detail later on).

When It Comes to Hydration, Go Deep and Go Often

Dewy, firm skin is the most sought-after beauty trait in South Korea. While Western society may tend to focus more on achieving a matte complexion,

Korean women prep and prime their skin so that they are luminous and glowing. Dewy is the opposite of oily, though—it's a fresh look, not a greasy one.

In addition to their daily and nightly routines, many South Koreans hydrate with facial mists and moisturizers several times throughout the day and combat drying air with humidifiers (which are frequently well-designed and almost art objects). For more concentrated hydration as needed, sheet masks and sleeping packs are used to give skin (and the person wearing it) a little pick-me-up.

It's About Brightening, Not Bleaching

A bright glow is the end goal in your skin-care game. A lot of Korean skin-care products are labeled "whitening," but this actually means "brightening." Bright skin looks like it's lit from within, and South Koreans love to enhance brightness with a little makeup hack. In other words, highlighters are a dewy girl's best friend.

Most Korean "whitening" products are safe for people of all skin tones to use and don't have actual bleach in them. Most contain arbutin (an extract from bearberry or mulberry leaves) in them, which is a natural ingredient that inhibits melanin production. However, it's always a good rule of thumb to check the labels!

Skin Care Is Not Just a Luxury

Thanks to picky consumers and widespread demand, even the most innovative Korean skin-care products are usually affordable. There are skin-care shops on every corner (and even in the subway stations), so good skin is accessible to everyone, and you don't have to automatically assume that it comes with an out-of-your-budget price tag. You can get effective ingredients and cutting-edge formulas—all wrapped in luxurious packaging—and still pay your rent.

No Routine Is One-Size-Fits-All

You will rarely find two people with the same skin-care routine. Even the most popular, newsworthy products (the ones that show up on every blog) aren't for everyone, and what your best friend recommends wholeheartedly still might not work for you. Never feel pressured to blindly use products based on what you've heard, because every person's skin is unique and will react differently to variations in ingredients and formulas.

In Western cultures, we're taught to buy skin-care products according to how old, or "mature," our skin is, but that's an oversimplification. Instead of just looking at your age, you should analyze your skin and determine what conditions need to be treated.

Unfortunately, skin care is very much a trial-and-error process, and there really isn't a way to get it right the first time, nor can you just copy what someone else does and expect to see the same results. It's also important to know that your skin is continuously changing—because, you know, *life* happens.

Korean women understand this well. They've learned to recognize when a product is working for them. If it's not, they're quick to chuck it out without a second thought, cute packaging be damned.

Take Ownership of Your Skin—and Have Fun!

Your skin does not have to be a mystery. You can be in control of your skin, and you don't have to wake up every morning wondering what might have appeared overnight. Yes, this is going to take a little time and effort on your part, but it doesn't have to be drudgery. This is pampering, not cleaning the kitchen.

When I was first learning about skin care, I was lucky enough to have so many local skin-care gurus (my new Korean friends, mainly) teach me how to get started with a legit, multistep routine. While at first it seemed like a lot of products, I was surprised that my regimen didn't take more than ten minutes in the morning and at night. A lot of the steps were just something I did once or twice a week.

I enjoyed pampering my skin on my own terms, and it felt great that I could be so knowledgeable about something that once left me clueless. When I'd travel to a new city with a different climate or get stressed over work deadlines, my skin might freak out, but I didn't. I really got to know my skin, which was crucial to maintaining it as well. And it wasn't a chore. My routine quickly became the highlight of my mornings and evenings, and it wasn't long before I began to recognize what I needed to use and what products were right for me.

And who am I kidding? I was hooked when I saw the results. My dull, dry skin was starting to look brighter and more supple, and my skin tone was more even and clear. My fine lines and pores were less visible, and I felt like I was taking off all those extra years I'd added at the beach. My skin felt dewy to the touch.

Any suspicions I had about the improvements being all in my head and not on my face (aka the placebo effect) were erased when I went home for the holidays. People complimented me on how good my skin looked, which never used to happen, and I couldn't help it—I glowed.

SKIN STORIES: Young Ah Kim

CREATIVE DIRECTOR OF CROSSPOINT NEW YORK, A GLOBAL BRANDING AND DESIGN FIRM THAT WORKS WITH TOO COOL FOR SCHOOL, MOON-SHOT, DR.JART+, INNISFREE, AND LANEIGE

The Korean cosmetic industry is very competitive. Companies are always searching for ways to differentiate themselves. Packaging is one way to stand out because it makes products eye-catching and can give the user a better overall experience. The quality of the products is obviously important, and though Korean companies typically do not substitute quality for packaging, they know very well the value of good packaging and make sure it doesn't fall to the wayside.

A product is more valuable the more unique it is, and Korean brands have to be unique to survive in the ultracompetitive market. I think Koreans are early adopters—they love trying the latest and greatest—which is why so many products are repackaged or renewed after just one or two years, or presented in limited edition sets.

With Too Cool for School, customers start to experience the brand from the moment they walk into the store. There is so much thought and effort put into the decor. It's designed from floor to ceiling. So it's not just the product packaging but also the shopping experience. It almost feels like you're transported to another world. We want it to be inspiring and fun and to give our customers a whole new experience—something for everyone and something they haven't seen before.

This doesn't just apply to cosmetic shops, but all manner of Korean retail businesses. The visual experience is emphasized wherever you go. Step into a coffee shop, and you'll notice the detail of the decor was painstakingly planned to provide the optimal ambiance for a good coffee shop. It's almost as if the visual atmosphere makes the coffee taste better. There is a strong culture of visual design and branding in Korea. We're lucky to be a part of that.

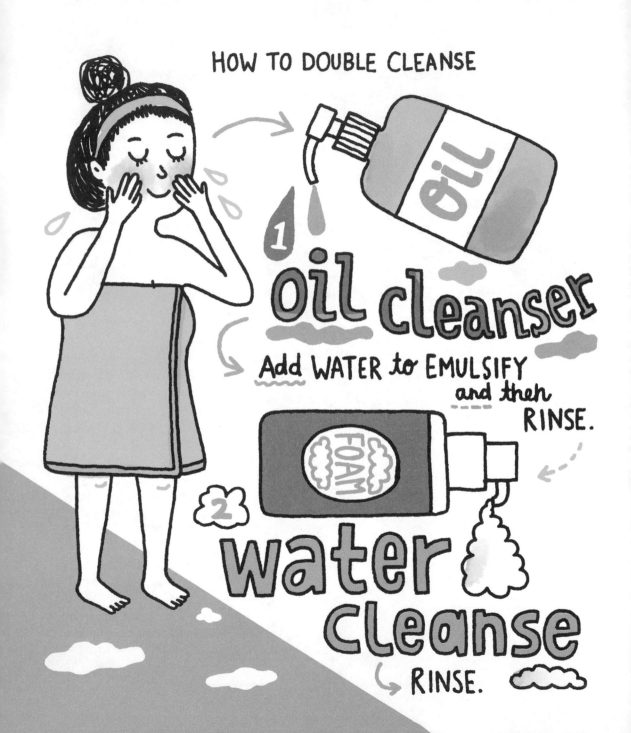

The Double Cleanse:

Cleansing So Nice, You Do It Twice

When I moved to Seoul, I started to learn new things almost instantly. For example, how to down several shots of soju at a company dinner and still make it to work in the morning, how to address my elders, and how to use a bidet (and like it).

All of this was to be expected. What I didn't anticipate was that I'd also learn how to wash my face. I mean, what? I'd already been doing it for ten years, which should be more than enough experience. How hard can soap and water be?

But that's just it right there: While the right way to wash your face isn't actually hard, it *is* about more than just soap and water.

As you no doubt know by now, skin care is cumulative. There's no one single trick that will transform your skin overnight; instead, the condition of your skin is determined by how you treat it, day in and day out, over the span of months and years. That said, we're all looking for a bit of instant gratification, so if you want your face to look better ASAP, change the way you wash it. No lie—as soon as I did, my skin looked clearer and felt softer within a week.

Skin-Care Crimes and Misdemeanors

Before I moved to Korea, I'd always considered cleansing one of the least important steps in my already suspect skin-care routine. Cleanser was meant to be washed off, and it was on my skin for only a few seconds at most—why not skimp on this step and save on time and money? Better to invest in moisturizers and creams that stayed on my face for hours—surely, that was where skin care really counted.

But no: Cleansing is not only the first step of your skin-care routine, but it's also the foundation. It's what sets the stage for the efficacy of everything else you use. Now that I know this, I pay extra-close attention to it, and I am willing to spend a little more time and money to make sure I'm selecting the right products for not just cleansing, but for cleansing the right way.

When I started talking to my friends about cleansing, I learned that I was far from alone in not knowing how to really wash my face. A lot of them admitted to not giving it much thought, and others copped to flopping in bed at night without washing their faces at all. And I get it—we've all been there on nights when we've had a few drinks, or are just otherwise exhausted, and the thought of spending even five more minutes awake to wash your face is just . . . *zzzzzzzz*. But taking the day to bed with you isn't just bad for those with oily or acne-prone skin; it's bad for everyone.

As I mentioned before, your skin is your largest organ, but you might be shocked to find out just how large: It makes up 10 percent of your total body weight (kind of gross but also awe-inspiring to think about). The primary function of your skin is to act as a barrier between the inside of your body and the rest of the world: It keeps the water in and all the impurities (such as allergens, microbes, and pollutants) out.

Going to bed without washing your face can lead to congested pores and acne breakouts. Makeup, sebum (an oily, waxy substance that is secreted by your sebaceous glands to protect the skin), and environmental impurities like pollution can settle into your pores, making them appear larger and causing blackheads (though they're dark in color, blackheads aren't actually trapped dirt, but a mixture of dead skin cells and sebum that oxidizes and darkens when it's exposed to air). Add a little bit of bacteria to this face sludge, and you get inflammation and an infection—a good old-fashioned zit.

#SoKoSecret: No matter what you do, don't pick or try to squeeze the zit. The bacteria that are living in your follicles may rupture and spread to other follicles if you forcefully squeeze it, which can cause more breakouts!

You certainly knew that not washing your face can cause pimples, but I'm about to drop another bomb: It can also accelerate aging. The grime that collects on the skin throughout the day contains free radicals, which—in spite of their awesome name—do some pretty not awesome things to your skin. They disrupt and kill skin cells, which in turn cause the breakdown of natural elastin and collagen (the components of your skin that keep it firm and plump) and creates wrinkles. Not thoroughly washing free radicals off at night gives them even more time to do their damage.

Air pollution is a big source of free radicals, and skin care that combats the harmful effects of daily pollution exposure is one of the next big frontiers for many Korean beauty companies. Pollution is a growing concern worldwide, but women in Asia have particular reason to be concerned.

#SoKoSecret: To reduce free radical damage, you can apply antioxidants topically or consume them. Some of the popular ones are green tea and vitamins A, C, and E, so keep those on your radar.

Spend enough time strolling Korean beauty aisles (or enough time watching *Get It Beauty*) and you'll begin to see the word "dust" pop up a lot. This isn't referring to the bunnies that gather under your bed, but "yellow dust," an Asian weather phenomenon in the spring in which clouds of desert dust from China blow across Japan and Korea.

Yellow dust also carries a ton of harmful pollutants, which is why you'll see people in Seoul wearing face masks on days when warnings are issued. If you don't, you can smell it in your nose, taste it in your mouth, and feel the grit on your skin. Air pollution is still much more extreme in China, but it's a growing problem everywhere, and seven out of the ten most polluted cities in the United States are in California. If I can't get you excited about washing your face, at least I can scare you into it.

Introducing the "Double Cleanse"

Cleansing and cleansing *thoroughly* are two very different things. Splashing water on your face and rubbing it with a towel is not cleansing at all (sorry, dudes).

Korean women are obsessed with how to properly cleanse their skin because they know it's the first step toward the final goal: a dewy, soft glow. Neglecting their cleansing routine would be akin to blasphemy. For many Korean women, a proper cleanse is a double cleanse, which means a first round with an oil-based cleanser, then a second with a water-based one. Now, I know, I know: You're probably thinking, *You're telling me that not only do I have to wash my face every night, but that I have to do it twice?*

All this double cleanse business isn't just a "Korean thing." We spent a long time discussing the double cleanse in my esthetician classes, and a lot of stateside dermatologists recommend it, too. The old California Charlotte neglected to wash her face before going to bed a few too many times, but now I actually look forward to the time that I spend taking off my makeup and city grime every evening.

Now, I know that sounds like something only an OCD person would say, but trust me, my friends (and husband) would vouch that I'm one of the least anal people they know. It's just that I've learned to treat cleansing, and my entire skin-care routine, as a way to unwind after a stressful day. If I fail to wash up (like that time I forgot to bring a cleanser on vacation), I fall asleep with a nagging feeling that I left something unfinished. I can feel my makeup partying it up in my pores like a kid whose parents went out of town.

So hear me out! If a double cleanse sounds like one too many, think about it this way: If you're going to spend time and attention putting your face on in the morning, doesn't it deserve the same care to remove it at night? If you truly want to get all that gunk off your face (and I'm sure you do), a double cleanse is the way to do it. Here's how:

Remove Your Eye and Lip Makeup

If you don't wear eye makeup, you'll skip this step, but eye and lip makeup are the most stubborn to remove (and also the stuff most likely to smear on your pillow), so they're the top priority. If I'm wearing more eye makeup than usual, or especially if I'm wearing waterproof mascara, I'll soak a cotton round with makeup remover, then place it on one closed eye and let it sit there for a good ten to fifteen seconds. If you use cotton swabs, hold the soaked swab in place for a few seconds at a time as you work your way around your eyes.

In the past, I've made the mistake of just rubbing the soaked cotton all over my eyes and immediately cleansing, then wondering why my eyeliner didn't budge. When you've got long-lasting makeup on, you really need the remover to mingle with the oil-based products for a while so that it breaks them down and they become easier to remove. Give it time and treat it gingerly, especially when it comes to the skin around your eyes, which is the thinnest and therefore the most prone to wrinkle. The more easily your makeup comes off, the less likely you are to pull and tug at your skin.

You should look for an oil-based makeup remover, and if you're using one that stings or otherwise irritates your eyes, chuck it now! Stinging is never a sign that something is "working"; it's a sign that your body doesn't get along with it. Also, if you're a contact lens wearer, take them out first.

The First Cleanse: The Oil Cleanser

Oil cleansers aren't bad, they're just misunderstood! In Western skin care, we're often taught to shy away from anything with the word "oil" in it for fear of clogged pores and acne. The reality is, though, that oil cleansers can actually be a godsend for oily, sensitive, and acne-prone skin.

Basic science rules apply here: Oil laughs in the face of water. Think of a parking lot on a rainy day: You can see oil pool on top of puddles, but it doesn't dissolve. But oil likes oil, so an oil cleanser can help break down and remove excess sebum and oil-based impurities like makeup, silicones, and sunscreen.

I was first introduced to oil cleansers when a generous friend in Korea gave me one as a gift. I remember clumsily slathering the oil on my face, and at first I didn't like it at all. I felt like I was adding oil to my face, rather than removing it. But the instant I rinsed it off, I was hooked. My face was far from an oil slick. It felt cleaner and softer and even looked brighter. Over the next few months, I carefully rationed the contents of that bottle, convinced this was so good that it had to be a secret. When I finally discovered that every beauty line in Korea makes its own oil cleanser, my hoarding was replaced with total promiscuity. I wanted to try them all.

Now, not a morning or night goes by when I don't use an oil-based cleanser (I take oil cleansing cloths with me when I travel). In the morning, you're not using an oil cleanser to remove makeup, but you still want to get rid of all the sebum and sweat that built up overnight, as well as any leftover nighttime skin-care products. For one thing, it's kind of fun, because you dispense it in your palms and then slide it over your face, which feels great. When doing so, spread it evenly over your entire face using your fingertips and gentle, circular motions.

#SoKoSecret: You can use natural oils like castor or coconut oil to oil cleanse, but they're more likely to leave behind an oily residue. It's better to use specially formulated oil cleansers that are designed to emulsify and wash off easily with water.

After I've thoroughly massaged the oil cleanser all over my face, I add a splash of lukewarm water to emulsify it. Though they sound very simple, a lot of technologies go into making oil cleansers so effective, and they usually are not 100 percent oil. When mixed with warm water, most are designed to turn milky and wash off very easily (cold water won't really do the job).

There aren't a ton of oil cleansers in the Western skin-care market just yet, but that is quickly changing. My current favorite cleansing oils are the ones that come in solid form, which means the oil doesn't drip down your arms or all over the bathroom sink. You just scoop a bit into your palms and then rub your hands together to liquefy it. Voilà! Most of these are also the kind that emulsify with warm water.

Multitask with a Face Massage

While you're cleansing and your fingers are able to slip and slide with ease, you can add in a minute or two of facial self-massage and take the benefits of washing your face even deeper. Massaging your face promotes blood circulation and can contribute to a healthier glow, not to mention that it just feels good.

Think of your blood as your body's own GrubHub: It's what carries nutrients from your heart to all the other parts of your body. The deeper levels of your skin contain tiny blood vessels, but the top layer contains none at all, so when you give your face a massage, you're helping to give that tiny bit of circulation a little boost. This is especially important in the winter and in colder climates, as circulation to your skin decreases in frigid weather, contributing to seasonal dry skin.

When you massage your face, you want to work with the direction of the muscles, not against it. Starting just underneath your cheekbones, use the knuckles of your first two fingers (with your hands in fists) and work out and slightly up from there. Press as firmly as what feels good to you, since the oil will keep the pressure from pulling your skin.

Then, still using your knuckles, trace them up the sides of your nose to the top of your forehead, then down along the perimeter of your face. Finally, use the pads of your fingers to lightly massage under your eyes, as this can help drain puffiness. Start at the bridge of your nose and move out to your temples.

When you're done, wash the oil off with warm water, then pat your face dry. Let me repeat: *pat pat pat* instead of an up-and-down scrubbing motion that pulls your skin every which way. You don't want to vigorously move your face up and down, as this could lead to wrinkles.

To be honest, there isn't a ton of scientific data about repeated facial motions leading to wrinkles because it's hard to study. Since wrinkles don't develop overnight, you'd have to maintain a controlled environment for twenty years or more to properly measure the results. But I believe it, and it turns out that once again, this was an area where my mother knew best. I have a habit of scrunching my nose when I laugh. Whenever my mother would catch me in the act when I was younger, she'd scold me and tell me to stop. I didn't pay any attention, but now when I look in the mirror, I can't help but think that Mom was right: Crinkles lead to wrinkles, and there they are, right across my nose.

The Second Cleanse: The Water-Based Cleanser

This step is probably familiar to you. After you've washed with your oil cleanser, follow with a water-based one to banish any sweat, dirt, or water-based debris that's still hanging around.

For this step, you can use a gel or foam cleanser—whatever you prefer and feels best on your skin. When you're using a water-based cleanser, it doesn't matter what temperature the water is, and here's a secret: A cleanser that foams isn't necessarily any better than one that doesn't. Foaming doesn't increase a cleanser's effectiveness or provide any extra benefits. Beauty companies just make cleansers foam to give people what they want: bubbles, lots and lots of bubbles.

Two Little Letters About Cleansing: pH

So now you know *how* to wash your face, but what do you use to do it? Because cleansers are an essential part of your skin care, choosing the right product is important, and it's about a lot more than just what is going to look good on your bathroom counter. It's about science and, specifically, pH.

Understanding pH can be a bit complicated, but once you've got a handle on it, finding a cleanser with the right pH for you is easy. pH ranges from 0 to 14, and this number indicates a substance's ratio of acidity and alkalinity, with 0 the most acidic, 14 the most alkaline, and 7 neutral. In its healthiest state, your skin is slightly acidic, usually 5.5. If your skin is too acidic, it can be irritated, prone to breakouts, and very oily. If your skin is too alkaline, it can look dull, feel extremely dry, and become flaky. Balance is key here.

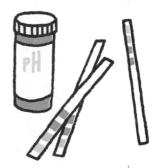

I used to love the feeling of tightness that came after I washed my face with that orange acne wash. You probably know that sensation—it feels as if your skin is cracking when you move. I used to interpret this as a sign that my cleanser was working, that my pores were tighter and even cleaner. But the truth is that tightness isn't a sign of skin being clean, but a sign of damage. Cleansers that are too alkaline overdry your skin, stripping it of its essential oils and natural moisture. Not only can this cause dryness and irritation, but it can also make your oil glands try to overcorrect by producing too much oil. So not what you wanted, right?

Our skin is topped with something called the acid mantle, a thin protective barrier made up of sebum and sweat. A lot of environmental factors (pollution, smoke, wind, water) can make the skin vulnerable because it breaks down the acid mantle, increasing your chances of developing skin conditions such as eczema and rosacea. A damaged acid mantle can even result in acne, because bacteria can penetrate much more easily when it's compromised, and flaky patches, because your skin can no longer retain its natural moisture.

INGREDIENT SPOTLIGHT:

Benzoyl Peroxide

Benzoyl peroxide is a common ingredient in acne treatments. It has antibacterial properties and can penetrate into the hair follicles to kill the bacteria that are causing pimples. Keep in mind, it can also sting your skin and overdry it, which could lead to redness, flaking, and other unwanted side effects.

This is why you need special soap for your face and can't just use that bar that's in the shower. In fact, your typical fragrant bar soap is highly alkaline (usually with a pH of around 8–10) and irritating for delicate facial skin and your body. On the flip side, a cleanser that is too acidic won't do much, because you actually need a slight alkalinity to properly dissolve dirt and be effective in cleansing. If you have normal skin, then the pH level of your cleansers isn't that big of a deal, but it's definitely something that people with acne-prone or sensitive skin should be aware of.

It's quite simple and inexpensive to check the pH of all your skin products (and it's also fun and kind of addicting). You can buy a whole bunch of pH strips for only a few bucks from Amazon, any big-box retailer like Walmart, or your local hardware store. Dip the strip in your cleanser or moisturizer and the colors will start changing quickly. After a minute passes, match it to the color pH guide that comes with the strips. (By the way, only water-based products will have a pH, so there's no need to test cleansing or moisturizing oils.)

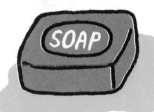

#SoKoSecret: The skin on your body is generally thicker (about 0.6 mm) and less sensitive than the skin on your face (0.12 mm), which is why it can tolerate a cleanser with a higher pH. However, you still want to be wary of soaps and body washes that leave your skin feeling too tight and dry, and always apply a moisturizer when you get out of the shower.

Tonering It Up

Now that you've done the double cleanse, it's time to break out the toner so you can, er, cleanse again?! Yes, but hear me out! This is your skin's pH we're talking about here, and well-formulated toners are designed to cleanse and reset your pH balance after using a very alkaline cleanser.

Advances in skin-care technology mean that fewer companies are making alkaline cleansers. So now toners focus on hydrating and fortifying the barrier to keep skin smooth and protected.

A toner by any other name is still a toner, and in Korea, the most popular ones go by several terms, including *activating serum, freshener, refresher, skin softener,* and even simply *skin.* All are very gentle and focus on protecting the acid mantle and providing hydration. They're normally chock-full of nutrients; humectants (such as glycerin), to help the skin retain moisture; and ceramides, to help skin cells bind.

You'll want to use toner as part of your morning and night routine (that is, every time after you cleanse your skin). Think of toner as prep school for your pores: It gives them a head start for what comes next and will help your skin absorb your skin-care products. Picture your skin as a dried-up sponge. If you try to put a heavy cream on it, a brittle, dry sponge won't accept it—it isn't "prepped" for moisture. But if you wet the sponge, the cream will sink in more easily. That's exactly why toners are a great addition to your skin-care routine.

I've used a wide variety of toners and I've learned to shy away from ones that are *astringents,* the term for formulas that contain a high percentage of witch hazel or alcohol. If you have oily skin you may actually enjoy the feeling of your skin being degreased, but don't fall into that trap. Alcohol inhibits the skin's ability to repair itself and even triggers more inflammation and acne.

Flashback to that eighty-dollar toner I bought from Bloomingdale's: It was so full of alcohol that it smelled like something from the first aid aisle at CVS, and brought me several bouts of breakouts and skin that seemed oilier. I finally tossed it, and for a long time I ditched toners altogether. But when my Korean friends taught me to be wary of any skin product with a high alcohol content, hydrating toners became my jam, and I haven't looked back since.

INGREDIENT SPOTLIGHT:
Alcohol

Products with denatured alcohol (usually just called alcohol) as a main ingredient are terrible for your skin because they can irritate it, damage the barrier, and produce free radicals. Don't confuse this with the good alcohols, like cetyl alcohol and stearyl alcohol (sometimes called "fatty alcohol"), which are often used as emollients and have beneficial effects.

Sometimes I like to transfer my toner into a spritz bottle and spray it all over my face and neck. Then I pat it in gently with my fingers, which lets all those hydrating and soothing ingredients soak in and gets your skin ready to ace what comes next. Check page 107 for a curated list of my favorite toners to find one that's right for your skin.

SKIN STORIES: Soo Joo Park

SUPERMODEL

I was born in Korea but grew up in suburban California. I wear a lot of makeup for work, so on my days off, I don't wear any. On these days, I clean two to three times with a foaming cleanser, sometimes using a vibrating wand brush. I rinse, spray on a bit of toner or use a coconut spray on a cotton pad, then apply moisturizer and a little bit of eye cream.

When I have work, that's a different story. I have to add a preliminary step of wiping the makeup off, so I apply Banila Co. Clean It Zero Classic, an oil cleansing balm that I massage into my skin. The heat of my hands melts the balm into a smooth liquid. It breaks down my makeup and makes it easy to wipe away with my Koh Gen Do makeup wipes. After cleansing, I begin my usual routine. These days I really like the Belif True Aqua Moisturizing Bomb. It's a gel cream that has a light, refreshing texture that absorbs quickly and doesn't leave me feeling sticky.

Sometimes I'll come home exhausted and fall asleep with my makeup on—which I wouldn't recommend to anyone.

Cleansing is important because having clean skin is crucial in maintaining a blemish-free and youthful face. Good personal hygiene can't hurt anyone.

Some nights I like to treat my skin to a sheet mask. I also try to pack a sheet mask when I know I'm going to be on a long flight, because the air is so dry on the plane. Hydration is important to keeping skin healthy and beautiful, so it can look good even without makeup. At the end of the day, my goal is to wear minimal makeup.

If I'm not working, but still feel like I should put in some effort, I'll go for some variation of no-makeup makeup. I make do with just concealer and a little blush on my cheeks. I don't usually wear bright lip colors, but I do make sure my lips aren't chapped. My favorite lip balm is actually the one they give out on Korean Air—Davi Napa. I also never leave home without oil blotters in my bag.

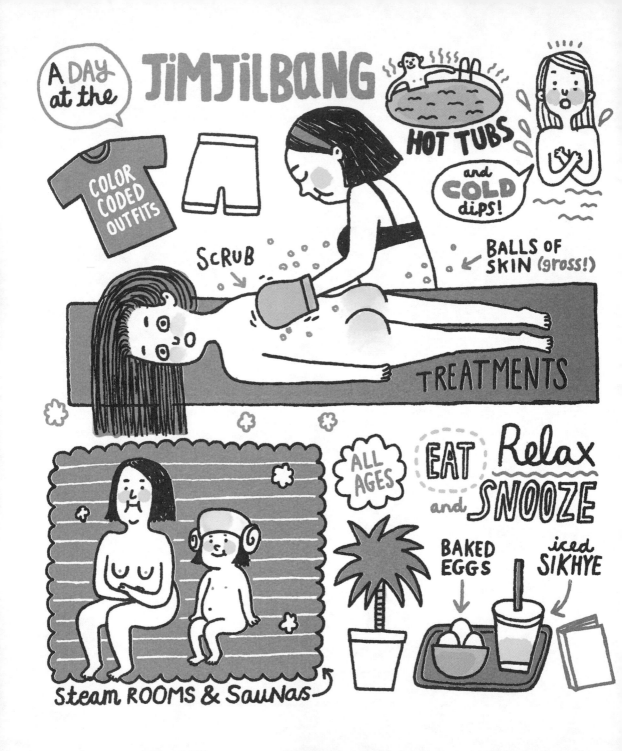

The Magic of Exfoliation

(and How to Be K-Spa Savvy)

When I was a kid, my mom would make it a point to use a rough cloth to scrub my entire body, but once my mosquito-bite boobs started to sprout, those weekly scrub downs were not welcome anymore. It was up to me to continue that tradition in the bathtub, but instead, I used what all my friends used, which was a nice, soft loofah and a big bottle of fruity body wash.

But after I started making trips to the sauna as an adult, a wimpy loofah wasn't enough. Now I use a washcloth to scrub from head to toe in the shower and have learned that exfoliating doesn't just feel good, but that it's actually good for you.

Let's get technical for a second. Your skin naturally sheds billions of skin cells a day, which actually contributes to dust. Gross, right? But if it doesn't shed properly, or if the shedding slows down, your skin can become dry and dull, and you may suffer from clogged pores and develop whiteheads, blemishes, and an uneven skin tone. This buildup of skin cells can even be the cause of those flaky skin flare-ups that are responsible for your makeup looking patchy and that can't even be tamed with moisturizer. Exfoliation gives your body's natural skin-cell shedding a boost and encourages cell regeneration, which results in a brighter and more even skin tone and smoother skin texture. You can exfoliate daily, weekly, or even just once a month, as it really depends on the condition of your skin.

Removing excess skin cells also helps your moisturizers and other products absorb more easily. Not having to fight through a layer of dead cells, your products can go straight to the epidermis, which ultimately means your skin will retain more moisture. The act of exfoliating can also help stimulate collagen production (to keep skin firm), improve circulation, and diminish the appearance of fine lines and wrinkles. If you've got oily or acne-prone skin, exfoliating helps clear away the dead skin cells that can get trapped in pores and cause blackheads and congestion.

Chemical or Mechanical: The Right Exfoliator for Your Skin

As we discussed before when talking about cleansers, the skin on your body is thicker than the skin on your face, so you don't want to go to town on your elbows and cheeks with the same vigor, or tools. Exfoliators mostly fall into two categories: mechanical and chemical. Mechanical exfoliation uses products such as sugar scrubs or brush bristles (such as a Clarisonic) for the face, or Korean moms armed with Italy towels for the body, to physically slough off dead skin cells from the surface of the skin. Mechanical exfoliation is good for normal to combination skin, but be cautious of using these methods if you have active breakouts or dry or sensitive skin.

#SoKoSecret: Skin that's frequently red, swollen, or itchy could have eczema. If you're experiencing eczema, stay away from both mechanical and chemical exfoliators and instead focus on moisturizing to protect the skin's barrier.

The downside here is that the physical nature of the mechanical exfoliation process can irritate skin, causing it to produce more oil and leading to more acne. If you have active pimples (such as those with a white tip), avoid mechanical exfoliators, as you don't want pimples to burst and spread bacteria to the surrounding skin.

Even without acne, you should still handle mechanical exfoliators with care. For example, if you're using an electric rotating brush, limit the amount of time and pressure you press the rotating brush on your skin. Also, be careful of what mechanical exfoliants are used, because if the material used to make the scrub isn't high quality, the rough, sharp edges of the granules can actually cause micro-tears in your skin.

In general, look for ingredients such as sugar, jojoba beads, or oatmeal, as all are fairly gentle on skin. Walnut and apricot scrubs, while popular,

The Magic of Exfoliation

have uneven and odd-shaped granules that can have sharp edges and spell bad news for your skin.

If you're using a rotating brush or exfoliating cloth for your face, you can use it during the second step of your double cleanse with your water-based cleanser. If you're using a separate exfoliating scrub, do your double cleanse, then use the scrub on wet skin, wash it off, and follow with your toner.

On the flip side, chemical exfoliation uses acids or enzymes to remove dead skin cells. Acids and enzymes break down and dissolve the lipids that act like glue and hold the dead skin cells together. Some acids can even work deep into pores to remove sebum, which is an extra bonus, because dead skin cells aren't just on the surface—they can settle deep into pores.

Acids used in chemical exfoliators are categorized as alpha hydroxy acids (AHA) and beta hydroxy acids (BHA). Some common AHAs include glycolic acid and lactic acid, and both can be found in skin-care products in concentrations from 5 to 15 percent. Starting at 12 percent, it's considered a chemical peel.

#SoKoSecret If you want something even gentler, enzymes (like bromelain and papain, which come from fruit) are an alternative to acids and digest the proteins between skin cells to help loosen up and sweep away dead ones.

Glycolic acid is a smaller molecule than lactic acid, so it penetrates into your pores very quickly, which can lead to irritation. Lactic acid is a larger molecule, penetrating more slowly, and is thus gentler than glycolic.

A popular BHA is salicylic acid, which is great for acne-prone and oily skin types because it breaks down oil and clogged pores and is anti-inflammatory and antibacterial. Most salicylic acid skin-care products can be applied and left on throughout the day if they have concentrations of 1 to 2 percent; anything higher than that should be rinsed off. Once again, moderation is key, as overusing salicylic acid can dry out your skin.

For chemical exfoliants, you'll want to apply them after washing your face and using your toner. Be careful to avoid the eye area, since this is extra-sensitive skin, and then follow with the rest of your skin-care routine in order. If you're using any retinols or prescribed products, double-check with your doctor to make sure that these products can be used together safely.

#SoKoSecret: Both glycolic and lactic acid have hydrating properties, which means you get to fight signs of aging and hyperpigmentation *and* plump up your skin while exfoliating. Bonus points.

Dead Skin: Your Body's Natural SPF

After you use chemical or mechanical exfoliators, you mustn't forget to moisturize! Exfoliation weakens your skin's barrier, and you want to re-hydrate and protect with a good moisturizer.

As important as it is to exfoliate, dead skin cells do act as your body's natural defense against the sun, and banishing them makes you extra sensitive to UV rays. You're more susceptible now to hyperpigmentation and sun damage, so it's incredibly important to regularly use at least an SPF 30 after you exfoliate. But let's be honest, you should be using an SPF every day regardless of whether you've exfoliated (more on that in chapter six).

Serious Exfoliation: Welcome to the World of Korean Spas

The spa is the cornerstone of Korean beauty culture. There are Korean spas (also known as K-spas) all over the world in major cities and suburbs with large Korean populations, and you can find them the same way you would a Western spa: get recommendations from friends and magazines, and read online customer reviews. However, the similarities might end there.

Even if you've never been to a spa, you've probably seen the experience portrayed in movies or on TV—you know, rich, snooty ladies sipping antioxidant beverages in near-total silence with cucumber slices over their eyes.

Now, to prepare yourself for a *jimjilbang*—the Korean word for spa, which roughly translates to "heated room"—throw all those ideas out the window. First off, a *jimjilbang* is very much a family and group affair, so you won't be wrapping yourself in a luxurious robe and retreating into solitude to the ambient noises of a birdsong CD. Instead, *jimjilbang*s are often multigenerational gathering spots where people go to get clean and chill out with their mothers, daughters, sisters, fathers, sons, brothers, cousins, friends, and even significant others. You're as likely to see a four-year-old at a Korean spa as you are a seventy-four-year-old.

Korean spas are also all day affairs. Instead of booking a treatment and then leaving as soon as it's over, you can eat, read, and snooze at the K-spa. And most are open twenty-four hours, so you can stay until the next morning.

If you're a total newbie and don't know what to expect, the K-spa can be a little jarring your first time (there's a lot of nudity involved, so you'll have to check your modesty at the door), but once you know what to expect, you'll likely become addicted.

Here, let me walk you through a day at the K-spa:

Checking In

Korean spas have separate areas for men and women, but also areas where everyone can hang out together. When you check in at one of these spas, you'll likely be given a key with a number that corresponds to the locker where you'll store your clothes and personal belongings, as well as a color-coded outfit to wear in coed areas. Men get one color and women get another, and these shorts and T-shirt combos fall someplace between pajamas and the gym clothes you wore in junior high. They're not cute, but they're comfortable, and that's the whole point.

The Shower

Once you're in the locker room, you'll change out of your street clothes, but don't put your spa clothes on yet. This is where the nakedness comes in. As soon as you're au naturel, you'll head to the showers, where you'll wash off before getting into any of the hot tubs or saunas. This helps ensure that the spa doesn't have hundreds of people a day bringing grime from the streets into the pools. You'll wash your hair, your face, and your body, and all thoroughly.

#SoKoSecret: Some spas provide shampoo, conditioner, and body wash. You can call ahead to see if you need to bring your own, or if you're particularly picky about products, you might want to do so anyway.

This is probably the part where you'll start to notice that nakedness is treated a little different from how it is in your gym locker room, where people try to change and shower as quickly as possible to minimize their time sans clothes. At the Korean spa, ladies will be walking around naked, having conversations naked, and even helping each other get clean—it's not uncommon to see friends or relatives standing butt naked and scrubbing each other's backs with exfoliating cloths.

Your first time, you'll probably feel a little shy, but hopefully this will fade as you see how comfortable everyone else is and as you settle into the fact that everyone is so into scrubbing their own limbs that they aren't paying you or your bits any attention.

The Wet Room

Tucked inside the locker room and still single-sex, the wet room will have tons of different pools and hot tubs. The hot tubs will likely have several different temperatures ranging from just lukewarm to piping hot, and some might have strategically placed jets for aqua-acupressure, to help relieve joint pain and enhance circulation. Some of the pools may even be filled with mineral or herbal treatments. A common one is the mugwort tea pool, which is said to help increase circulation and decrease inflammation.

The wet room will also probably have traditional dry saunas and steam rooms, as well as a cold plunge, which is a shock to the system that's supposed to get your blood flowing and help with lymphatic drainage.

Treatments and Body Scrubs

Most K-spas also offer treatments, ranging from massages to facials to classic body scrubs. The body scrub is one of my favorite things about Korean spa culture (it's the most hard-core exfoliation around), but again, it might be a bit of a shock if you hear the word "treatment" and think private room with scented candles.

If you've signed up for a treatment at a K-spa, you'll likely be asked to stay in the wet room until it's your time, and then someone will call your number or come find you.

The ladies (or men, for the guys) who perform the treatments are no-nonsense and usually dressed in uniform black underwear (nothing sexy: think maximum-coverage granny panties). Once they call your number, you'll proceed to the treatment area and lie down on a plastic-covered massage table.

As soon as you're lying down, they'll dump a bucket of warm water on you to start, then begin scrubbing you from head to toe. These scrubs are done with force and conviction and cover almost every inch. They will have you cock your knees open so that they can scrub your inner thighs, and while your modesty might cringe here, just remind yourself that they do this dozens of times a day and have seen it all before.

The Magic of Exfoliation

You'll be surprised to learn that you can actually see the dead skin cells being sloughed off, which roll off your back in gross little gray balls. It's disgusting, yes, but also highly satisfying. There's a sternness to a Korean body scrub as well, and to me, it always feels as if an aunt who has known me my entire life is simply scrubbing me down.

Most scrubs will conclude with a quick head and neck massage and a shampoo, and then you get up from the table feeling ten pounds lighter and with a shiny glow all over your body.

In case I haven't already made it clear, let me repeat myself: These scrubs are intense. I have a high threshold for pain, so they're not painful for me in the slightest, but every person is different. I've had friends with much more sensitive skin emerge bright red and on the verge of tears. The key here is to know

#SOKOSECRET: Most K-spas use Italy towels for these body scrubs. They're basically large mittens made of 100 percent viscose, and they come in bright colors. These towels are a Korean invention, but the fabric was first imported from Italy in the 1960s—hence the name. You can also buy your own Italy towels to use at home. They can be purchased for as little as a dollar each from Amazon or eBay.

what's right for you and communicate that to the lady in black undies. If something hurts, or she's scrubbing too hard, she won't know unless you tell her. Again, an important rule about the K-spa: Don't be shy!

The Family Room

After you're supersmooth from your intense body scrub, you'll put on your spa pajamas and head up to the communal coed rooms. Here, you'll see entire families, single people, and couples doing some serious lounging. They'll read comic books, watch dramas, gossip, or nap. One awesome thing about this room is that the floor is heated, so dozing off on a hard surface has never been so comfortable. It's not uncommon to see people snoring away, surrounded by chaos, directly on the floor, on a mat resting on a brick-shaped pillow, or in a reclining chair.

Many Korean spas have snack bars or full-on restaurants, so you can munch on everything from baked eggs to cold bowls of *naengmyun* (long, thin noodles in chilled broth) complete with *banchan,* an assortment of small, complimentary side dishes to sweet desserts like *patbingsoo* (red beans with shaved ice and condensed milk). At a lot of these places, your final bill is attached to your locker number, so you don't have to take cash or cards with you—you can just use your number and pay for everything at the end.

Here, there's no such thing as overstaying your welcome. In Korea, twenty-four-hour *jimjilbangs* are often a safe haven for salarymen and -women who stumble in too drunk to make the trek home before work the next morning, and these spas are especially popular in the winter, when people want to take maximum advantage of the heated floors.

The Dry Saunas

Around the heated floor, you'll see several doors that lead to different saunas. These range anywhere from 60°F to 200°F, and all promote resting, healing, and rejuvenation.

Each Korean spa will be different, but the sauna arrangement will likely be something like this: the salt sauna, full of said minerals to help with skin conditions; the jade sauna, supposedly good for reducing stress; the clay sauna, full of thousands of tiny clay balls that you can bury yourself in to be warmed from all sides; and the *bulgama,* which is like baking yourself in a clay pizza oven heated to more than 200°F. For all of these, you'll wear your spa pajamas, and you can stay as long as you want, though the recommended use is ten to twenty minutes. If you're new to saunas, start small and work up to a longer period of time. Also, keep in mind that heat affects everyone differently. If it makes you feel light-headed or dizzy, the *bulgama* might not be for you, even if there's an old lady happily snoozing away just a few feet from you. You can close your round of sauna-going with a stop in the ice igloo, which is a cold room said to firm the skin. It will also jolt you out of your overall Korean drama–*naengmyun*-sauna *jimjilbang* stupor and prepare you for your harsh return to the real world.

Korea's Communal Culture

· ·

When I first planned to move to Korea, my parents and friends at home worried that I'd be lonely. It turned out that they weren't right, but they weren't entirely wrong either.

In the beginning, I spent a lot of time alone in my little studio (also known as an "officetel," a portmanteau of "office" and "hotel" that refers to a residence in a multiuse building) near the company. I had plunked down quite a bit of cash (my meager life savings) to rent it, so I was forced to snag most of my furniture from expats who were selling it at majorly discounted rates when it was time for them to leave the country and return home.

My setup included a small, collapsible picnic table and bench that I used as my dining table and seating. One foot away from the dining table was my mattress, and right next to that was the kitchen. Let's just say that it wasn't in my best interest to cook anything that was particularly odorous, or else I'd run the high chance that my pajamas, hair, and socks would smell like last night's fried fish.

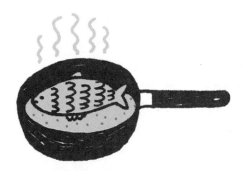

I quickly learned to avoid cooking fragrant dishes in the apartment, but it turned out to be not a huge deal at all. Korea's takeout options are on par with, if not exceed, Manhattan's. I could just order delivery, and in minutes, someone would bring fresh black bean noodles with all the side dishes in real dishware. After I was finished, I would leave the dirty dishes in a baggie outside my door, and the delivery guy would pick them up on his next round. It was hangover heaven.

Also similar to Manhattan, Seoul is so dense that stepping outside of my apartment meant I was seconds away from yummy bakeries, coffee shops, and convenience stores filled with snacks. Mom-and-pop restaurants that served home-style comfort foods were plentiful and inexpensive. Aside from a few fast-food dishes (such as In-N-Out, which I crave even now, since I live on the East Coast), I typically didn't hunger for anything non-Korean, because it was easy to find international food options: pizza, pasta, pad thai, and tacos that were, honest to God, just as yummy as they were stateside.

As I had expected, the Korean food was mouthwatering. Steamy and spicy stews, chewy rice cakes, and fresh veggie dishes were at my disposal—except for one thing: many of my favorite dishes were designed to be shared. Korean BBQ platters and spicy stews like *budae jjigae* could only be served if you were ordering family-style servings. Now, I could eat a lot, but BBQ for two was beyond my capacity.

I soon learned that food in Korea isn't the only thing meant to be shared, and there's a lot of value placed on spending quality time with your friends and family. It's why spas are designed to be all-ages affairs— why would you want to go somewhere if you couldn't take your daughter and your grandma with you?

Although I never cared about eating alone at a restaurant in the past, I suddenly felt awkward sitting by myself inside a bustling restaurant while groups around me shared drinks and platters of meat and pots of soup. This newfound awkwardness made me inhale my meals. I also became much more vigilant about planning meals with friends, so that I could work in some family-style dishes whenever I could.

My colleagues at work were always curious about how I was faring, because typically Koreans don't live in their own apartments until they go off and get married to start their own families. My early-twenties self, eating ramen alone in front of the TV, was actually totally fine with me—I'd been living independently since I was eighteen back home—but for many Koreans who learned of my plight, it seemed incredibly lonely.

Korea had always seemed very lovey-dovey to me, as it was not uncommon to see couples spooning as they slept in the *jimjilbang*, or cuddled up in a café corner and watching dramas on a shared iPad. But as I started to understand that most relationships had no privacy until the couple was married, this made total sense to me. It beats the hell out of hanging out with friends or your boyfriend at home, with your parents an earshot away from your high school angst.

I was also used to the get in, get out café culture in the United States, where asking for the Wi-Fi password is a shameful admission. However, Korean cafés didn't care if you lingered and actually encouraged it. Soon, the cafés were like my second living room and my preferred space to work, read, or catch up on e-mails.

Looking back, it was this communal side of Korean culture that I ended up embracing the most. My immediate family was not with me in Seoul, but my relatives and the new people I met made me feel as if I had always been part of their lives. It was clear to me that after about a year my work colleagues and I had *jeong,* which roughly means "playful affection," for each other. So when someone I worked with asked, "Why is your Korean still horrible?" or would tease me by saying, "Honestly, your date is too good-looking for you," I didn't get offended—they were treating me as if they were cousins I'd known my whole life.

Fortunately, whenever I get nostalgic for this cozy feeling, I can just make the trek to one of New York City's many Korean spas. Sure, there's probably no one there who will insult me because they like me so much, but I can still put on strange pajamas and nap on a heated *jimjilbang* floor, dreaming of *budae jjigae* and *hotteok* (sweet pancakes) in Seoul.

SKIN STORIES: India-Jewel Jackson

MANAGING EDITOR, HEARST MAGAZINES DIGITAL MEDIA

An afternoon at a Western spa is usually all about pampering and de-stressing, while an afternoon at a Korean spa is more about socializing. You go to lounge in the bath, catch up with your friends, and get a thorough cleansing simultaneously. I first discovered the Korean spa because I was searching for a twenty-four-hour spa in New York—I wanted to schedule a midnight massage for my mom to start her birthday off right. The only place I could find that offered this was a spot in Koreatown. After looking through the vast menu, I decided to go to the spa with her and have been hooked ever since!

My skin feels freakishly soft after a body scrub, and I love how squeaky clean I feel when they're done. Ironically, I hate how naked I have to be to experience it. I'll never feel comfortable walking around stark-naked in front of fifty strangers no matter how many times I go.

One thing: Whether you're visiting a Korean spa in New York City, Los Angeles, or Seoul, be prepared for the possibility of a language barrier, but it's unlikely to be an actual problem. Thanks to service menus and animated hand gestures, beauty is its own universal language. And it always works out in the end!

HOW TO properly SHEET MASK

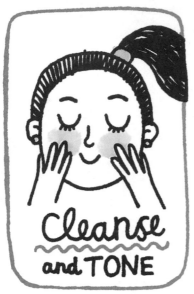

Cleanse and TONE

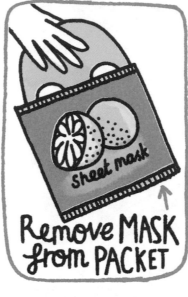

sheet mask

Remove MASK from PACKET

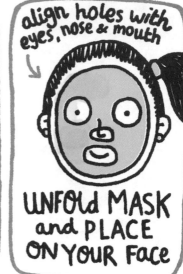

align holes with eyes, nose & mouth

UNFOLD MASK and PLACE ON YOUR FACE

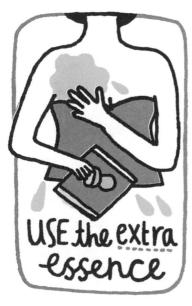

USE the extra essence

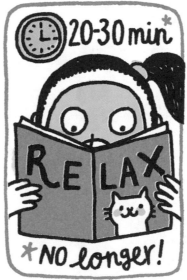

20-30 min*

RELAX

*NO longer!

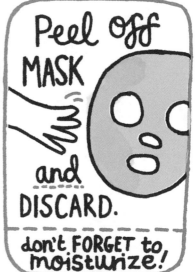

Peel off MASK and DISCARD.

don't FORGET to moisturize!

5

Chok Chok:

Moisturizing and the Art of Dewy Skin

Koreans love the dewy look so much that there's a phrase for it: *chok chok*. *Chok chok* doesn't just pertain to skin, but is used to describe something that is literally moist. While it's much desired in Korea, it's something that Western beauty has historically tried to cover up with mattifying primers, foundations, and powders—whatever kept the skin as matte as possible. But once you experience skin that is *chok chok,* you'll decide that it not only feels better; it looks better, too.

Glowy vs. an Oil Slick

· ·

In Seoul, I frequently met my friends for brunch in Garosu-gil, a popular treelined street with endless cafés, restaurants, and boutiques. Over a table covered with warm lattes and pastries, our conversations were the usual chitter-chatter: about the couple who broke off their engagement because of a bad reading from a fortune teller, the latest *mat-jib* ("delicious house," or highly praised restaurant), and, of course, our favorite topic, beauty. We swapped product recommendations as if we were Wall Streeters with stock tips, and sprinkled through our conversations were declarations of the next big thing: "I swear by this new cushion compact—it's so inexpensive and was sold out for weeks!" Also, talking about someone's *pibu* (the Korean word for "skin") was a crucial part of sizing them up: "He's dating this new girl. Have you seen her amazing *pibu*?"

Inevitably, someone would bring out a phone to illustrate her point, and at first I couldn't really wrap my head around what was causing so much talk and envy. Sure, so-and-so's ex-boyfriend's new girlfriend's skin looked amazing, but wasn't it just a tad too shiny? Last I'd checked, greasy was not in. Isn't that what they make oil-blotting papers for?

But the more time I spent in Korea, and the more women I observed, the more I realized that their foreheads weren't oil slicks, just glowingly moist. It was the opposite of matte—healthy, baby smooth, and radiant. For someone who spent the greater part of her life with a powder puff to her face, desperately blotting, I was now questioning everything I knew (about skin, at least).

I didn't want to jump on any bandwagon, but when I thought about *chok chok,* I could see why it would be the permanent future of skin and not just a passing fad. I'd been used to mattifying my face to the point of cracking, but when I started to pay attention and began using hydrating skin products, I couldn't just see the difference—I could feel it. My face felt fresh, and I no longer had to worry that the lower half would fall off if I laughed too hard at a joke.

At this point, you're familiar with cleansing, toning, and exfoliating, all of which are important pieces in the skin-care game. But the real game changer? Hydrating and moisturizing. Pretty much everything you've learned up to this phase is just a prelude, and those products were just the opening act. The headliners on your beauty counter are the ones that hydrate your skin and help it retain moisture.

If you're part of the YouTube generation like me (and even if you're not), it'll probably help to get a visual. So here it is: Think of your skin as your favorite leather shoe (I know, I know, but bear with me . . .). Without properly maintaining the leather with a polish, the leather will eventually start to crack or even start peeling. The shoe's texture will be rough and its color will be lackluster. No one—I repeat, no one—wants her face to look like an old leather shoe.

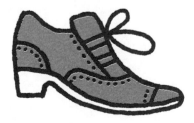

But your skin is actually similar to this leather in some ways: If you take care of it and keep it moist and supple, you'll see a difference over time. Without a seal to keep the moisture in and protect your skin, you'll really see life's wear and tear right there on your face.

Adding hydration to your skin plumps it up and fills in the gaps, which helps reduce the visibility of fine lines. No, this doesn't mean that you can slap on some lotion and see all your lines and wrinkles magically disappear, but lines will be more apparent on skin that is consistently dehydrated.

But let's set vanity aside for a moment and pretend you don't care about wrinkles: Moisturizing is still important because it helps keep your skin healthy. Without extra hydration, daily environmental exposures (especially those you're exposed to after you've stripped away your natural oils by washing twice a day) can cause tiny fissures in the outermost layer of the epidermis (the part of your skin called the *stratum corneum*) that make it more susceptible to bacteria and skin disorders. Your skin can become itchy, flaky, and irritated, and you might even see more acne crop up. Think of your stratum corneum as a tiny Fabergé egg (or brand-new iPhone): It's very thin and delicate, and you must protect it!

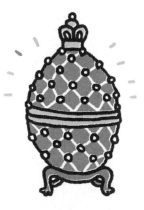

Day and Night Moisturizing:
This Is How You Do It

Unfortunately, you can't just splash your face with water and call it a day, as this can actually have the opposite of the desired effect and dry your skin out even more. Water molecules are too large to penetrate your skin, but are great at drawing water out of it. If our skin could really absorb water that easily, every time we took a shower we'd puff up like a blowfish—and let's all be thankful that doesn't happen.

Formulated moisturizers work because they hydrate the skin with ingredients that have smaller molecules to draw moisture to the skin and then retain it once it's there. And while dousing your face with water won't actually moisturize it, products are actually absorbed better when applied on a damp face.

Just as I explained in chapter three about the dry sponge vs. the damp sponge, it's beneficial to start with damp skin. I've gotten in the habit of applying my skin-care products right when I step out of the shower (before I even blow-dry my hair), and that really enhances the absorption of everything, from my toner to my night cream.

There is also an order in which you should apply your skin-care products, starting with the lightest consistency (such as liquid toners) and then moving toward the heaviest (like a rich cream). Applying the heaviest cream first would almost create an oily barrier that would make it harder for the others to penetrate. This is why most toners are formulated to be very watery, since they're one of the first products you apply.

Your Skin Deserves a Treat(ment)

But *wait*! Before you start tapping in that moisturizer, you might want to use a treatment product that's formulated to specifically target skin issues such as dullness, brown spots, redness, or fine lines.

Before you throw your hands up in the air and curse the beauty gods for sending you yet *another* step in your regimen, keep in mind that treatments are entirely up to you and what your skin needs. If your skin is in tip-top shape and you don't have any of the above concerns, bravo to you, and you can make the seamless move from toner to moisturizer. Even if you do decide to add a treatment to your morning or night routine, you don't have to use it every day.

In defense of yet another product, I do have to say that treatments are a huge part of the Korean skin-care routine, and most are used not just to treat, but to prevent. These skin-care products are the heart of the Korean skin-care routine, because they utilize the most powerful ingredients and are specifically designed to combat and lessen the signs of aging. Most of these products will be labeled as an essence, ampoule, serum, or booster. Let me break it down for you—it can be tricky to keep track!

Essences

Essences are a popular skin care category in Korea—many Korean people believe it is the heart of their regimen! Generally, essences have a thinner and more watery consistency than serums and ampoules, but most of them contain active ingredients to help hydrate, brighten, even out skin tone, firm skin, and reduce the visibility of wrinkles. You'll use these after toning and before moisturizing, and you'll pat them over your entire face.

Ampoules, Serums, and Boosters

Though products may be labeled as ampoules, serums, or boosters, all are generally used the same way and for the same range of purposes. They have a thicker consistency with a more potent concentration of ingredients (think of them as an essence reduction) and are frequently used as spot treatments, such as to target brown spots on your cheeks or fine lines around your mouth. They frequently come in glass bottles with droppers, so you can squeeze out only as much as you need. If you're adding one of these to your routine, you'll use it after your toner or essence, wait a few minutes for it to absorb, and then follow with your moisturizers. If you're using a treatment that increases sun sensitivity (like something with retinol), you might want to use it only as part of your nighttime routine to avoid UV exposure.

Treatments are one of the most personalized parts of a skin-care routine, so you might want to try a few different things, or get a consultation from a knowledgeable friend or esthetician, to find a product that is right for your specific needs and your skin type.

#SoKoSecret: Beauty companies are constantly blurring the lines between all four treatment products (essences, ampoules, serums, and boosters) making it increasingly difficult to define them. It's up to you to read the major ingredients to see what the product will do for you.

Your Personal Hydration Station

There are a plethora of moisturizers at your disposal to increase hydration and get you that much-desired *chok chok*. Deciphering what a moisturizer does for you, and which is right for you, often comes down to texture and function. Moisturizers usually contain humectants, which both prevent the loss of moisture and attract it to the skin, and/or lipids, which improve hydration and make skin smooth. Algae, hyaluronic acid, glycerin, sodium PCA, sorbitol, and propylene glycol are common humectants. As their names would imply, phospholipids and glycosphingolipids are lipids.

A moisturizer by any other name is still a moisturizer, but different types and formulations do different things and target different skin concerns. And while moisturizing should always be a part of your routine, you might want to use different products in the morning from those at night.

Emulsions

This term is used to describe a mixture of two or more liquids that are not entirely mixable—think oil and vinegar for salad dressing, or, in this case, oil and water for your skin. Most beauty lines in Korea include an emulsion, which is typically a light moisturizer formulated with tiny droplets of oil suspended in a water base. Since emulsions are so light, they are recommended for oily and combination skin types.

Lotions

An in-between moisturizer, a lotion is heavier than an emulsion and lighter than a cream. Most lotions are suitable for all skin types.

Creams

A cream is usually more oil than water, which means it is very rich and emollient. Many creams are formulated with skin-repairing ingredients to lock in moisture and nourish the skin while you sleep, which is why so many creams are marketed for use at night. Creams are good for dry and aging skin types.

Gel Creams

Gel creams absorb quickly and are lightweight because they are water based, which helps minimize clogged pores. These creams are great for hydrating oilier skin that is prone to breakouts and acne.

Facial Oils

Facial oils are used after toning or exfoliating and are applied directly on the skin. You can also add a few drops to your regular face lotion to up its powers when your skin is feeling especially dry or flaky. In general, facial oils aren't recommended for oily skin types.

Sleeping Packs

A sleeping pack, sometimes called a sleeping mask, is not a cloth mask that you use to cover your eyes while you get some beauty sleep. In the Korean beauty world, it's a product you use once or twice a week in the evenings (in place of your night cream) to give your skin a spa day's worth of hydration. Depending on the product, a sleeping pack can also help make skin brighter or firmer. You put it on like lotion, spreading a thin layer across your entire face, but unlike a night cream, you won't pat it in. Your skin will slowly absorb its hydration while you sleep, and then you wash it off in the morning. Sleeping packs are usually formulated with a gel-like consistency and go on clear, so don't worry—it won't look like you're sleeping with frosting on your face. You will want to try to fall asleep on your back, but most sleeping packs aren't really as messy as they might sound, so it's NBD if you toss and turn a bit during the night.

In Korea, "sleeping beauty" is a huge product category. During the day, your skin is working to protect the rest of your body, and then it repairs itself at night. It does most of its restoration between 10 P.M. and 4 A.M., so you'll see maximum benefit from any hydrating products you use during these hours.

#SoKoSecret: Still dry and tight even with the right moisturizer? Like most Korean households, invest in a humidifier that will add moisture to the air.

Sheet Masks

Sheet masks are one of the most popular and well-known beauty products to come out of Korea, and I've separated sheet masks from the essences and sleeping masks because they're a stand-alone beauty innovation.

Everyone and their mom are using sheet masks in Korea. You'll be hard-pressed to find a household without a sheet mask handy, and they've quickly become one of my favorite ways to pamper myself. These face masks are not to be confused with the paper nose and mouth coverings doctors wear when seeing a patient, or that people use on days when dust levels are high. Those are precautionary hardware. Sheet masks are beauty superstars.

Sheet masks are shaped to fit your face, with eyes, nose, and mouth cutouts, and they're drenched in the kind of active ingredients you would find in a bottle of essence. Most make you look like Jason from *Friday the 13th* (and provide infinite selfie opportunities), but you can also find them in colors, patterns, or even a pig or dragon face.

The two most popular kinds of sheet masks are made out of a cotton-type material (microfiber) or gel (hydrogel). Most hydrogel sheet masks are 100 percent water soluble, making it extra hydrating for your skin.

When it comes to getting that dewy glow, I find sheet masks to be the most effective. They work so well because while the sheet rests on your face, it acts like an icebreaker at an awkward party and forces the antioxidants and vitamins to mingle with your skin. With a lot of the skincare products you put on your face, some of the ingredients will evaporate before they even have the chance to penetrate your epidermis, but a sheet mask helps lock the nutrients in. Peeling it off is somewhat of an unveiling, and you'll see your face brighter, softer, and hydrated to perfection.

Sheet masks are relatively inexpensive, and the fun is in the variety. Think about winter, when cold winds and your heater on full blast severely dehydrate your skin. That's when you reach for a sheet mask with hyaluronic acid to bind moisture to the skin and antioxidants, such as vitamin C, to fight free radical damage and provide cell-communicating

Chok Chok

ingredients that help diminish the appearance of fine lines. In the middle of the summer, you can grab one to nourish the skin or to help treat breakouts. Sheet masks can be labeled by their specific ingredients (everything from blueberries and vitamin C to collagen and snail mucin) or by the skin conditions that they target. Whatever it is you're looking for, though, you'll find it, and it's unlikely that you'll leave the store with just one.

INGREDIENT SPOTLIGHT:
Snail Mucin

Snail mucin is not the oozy, gooey slime that you may think it is. It's an extract packed with nutrients such as hyaluronic acid, glycoprotein enzymes, antimicrobial and copper peptides, and proteoglycans—all ingredients commonly used in beauty products and proven to be beneficial to the skin. These ingredients have been known to stimulate the formation of collagen and elastin (that is, they're antiaging), repair damaged skin, and restore hydration, which has made snail mucin skin-care products very popular in Korea. (Snails are not harmed in this process!)

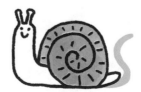

Companies are now making sheet masks for all sorts of body parts. You can find ones that treat ashy elbows or firm your boobs and butt (I'd say no selfies on these kinds of sheet masks, but maybe that's just me).

#SoKoSecret In Korea, they take "selcas," which is a portmanteau of the English words "self" and "camera." Common selca poses:

1. Hand on cheek to make face look slightly smaller
2. Puffing out cheeks to look endearing or cute
3. Selfie with stickers

Now share or post!

When I lived in Korea, I had the luxury of cheap weekly facials, but if you keep up with your skin-care routine at home by using sheet masks and other effective products, then you can frequently forgo the facials, which are definitely not cheap here in the United States. It's entirely up to you how often you use sheet masks—they're great for when you have twenty minutes to spare. Use them in lieu of your regular treatment, after cleansing and before moisturizing, once or twice a week, and in winter, when my skin feels extra tight and dry, I up that to about two to three times.

When it's hot or humid out, you can pop a sheet mask in the fridge so that when you're ready to use it, it's instantly cooling. Traveling? Bring one on an overnight flight so that your skin is charged up when you land. Big event where you have to look glowing? No need to rush off to an expensive facial to get a hydration boost—a sheet mask can let you do it in the comfort of your own home, and from anywhere between $1 to $10. Once you start, you'll find yourself a big believer in the sheet mask lifestyle, extolling the virtues of sheet masks to anyone who'll listen.

Since sheet masks are fun and relatively cheap, they're a great gateway into the world of skin care. So if you have a boyfriend who washes his face with the dish soap or a best friend who thinks SPF is NBD, slip them a sheet mask. You could be introducing them to a whole new world.

A QUICK SHEET MASK HOW-TO
(IN CASE YOUR INSTRUCTIONS ARE IN KOREAN)

After double cleansing and toning (see chapter three):

1. Tear open the pouch at the top and pull out the mask. The mask will be dripping wet—have a towel handy to wipe up the drips.

2. Sometimes masks will come with a plastic backing; don't forget to remove it. Unless the brand specifically mentions what side of the mask you should place on your face, it shouldn't matter what side you use. Unfold the mask and place it on your face, aligning the holes with your eyes, nose, and mouth.

3. Apply the excess essence in the pouch and the mask to your neck, shoulders, and hands. Those essences are good for your skin, so don't let any go to waste!

4. Take a power nap, read a book, swipe left or right, or simply zone out for about twenty to thirty minutes.

5. When you're ready, just peel off the mask and discard it. There's no reason for you to wash off the essence that is left behind, because it is good for your skin! When you look at your skin in the mirror, it should look brighter and

slightly plumper from the moisture it just absorbed. Also, touch it. Touch it! It should feel velvety smooth and, dare I say, *chok chok*?

6. Finish off the routine with a moisturizer (and SPF if you're heading out).

SKIN STORIES: Kim Ju Won

SHEET MASK EXPERT AND CEO OF IM1NE, A MASK MANUFACTURER

Sheet masks started becoming popular in Korea about a decade ago. Now they're a standard product offering for every skin-care brand in Korea and even the rest of Asia. There are more than eight hundred varieties of sheet masks on the market now. The most common types are hydrogel—which are 100 percent soluble, so that they slightly melt from the heat of your skin when they're on your face—and microfiber.

Sheet masks became such an important part of skin care because there was a desire for a product that would effectively hydrate and moisturize, but in a convenient way so that anyone could do it at home.

Your skin's barrier is made out of natural lipids, and one of the most important functions of skin care is to protect it. When the barrier is damaged, moisture can escape through tiny fissures in the skin, and this can cause flakiness and irritation. Sheet masks are one way to deliver intensive hydrating ingredients to the skin. If you use them consistently two or three times per week, you'll notice a difference in elasticity and a reduction in fine lines.

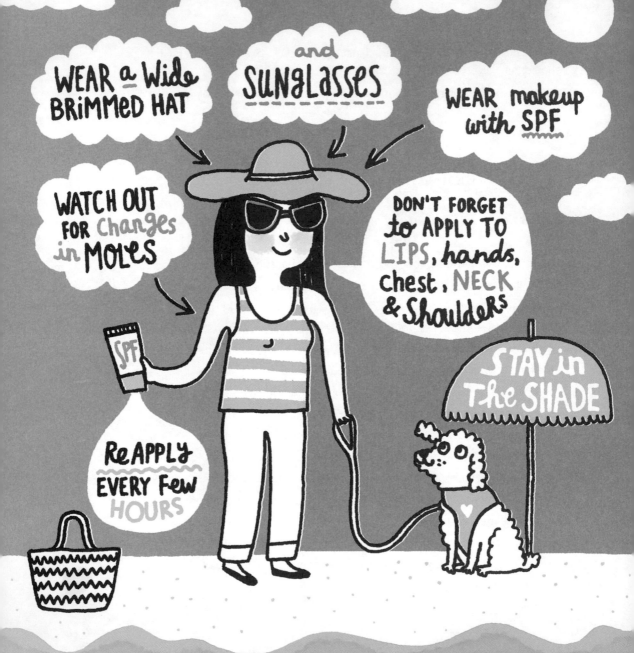

6

Sunscreen:

The Most Important Word in Skin Care

Oone word: "sunscreen." Did your eyes glaze over? I don't blame you. I'll be the first one to admit that, when it comes to skin-care topics, sunscreen is both confusing and boring. Makeup, sheet masks, oil cleansers—all kinda sexy, right? But sunscreen, well, it sounds about as exciting as homework.

So, on that note, I'm dedicating an entire chapter to it! But hey, I'm not doing this for my health; I'm doing it for yours—when it comes to sunscreen, we're not just talking about preventing premature aging, we're talking about preventing skin cancer. Everything we've previously covered—cleansers, toners, exfoliators, treatment products, and moisturizers—are ways to maintain and correct the damage that's already been done to your skin. Sunscreen's the last step, but probably the most important one, because now it's all about prevention, baby. (Did I make it sound sexy there? Well, I tried.)

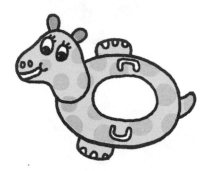

A Marathon, Not a Sprint

No matter what a commercial or label promises, there's no skin-care product that will result in dramatic, lasting improvements overnight. But even if you're not expecting immediate gratification, sunscreen is a product that will *truly* test your patience. Its purpose is to protect your skin, not improve it, and I think that's one of the reasons it's so hard to keep up with. Use it day in and day out, and you're not going to look better, just the same. But just think about that: If you can keep your skin looking pretty much the same, and minimize its damage and deterioration, that's no small feat over time. Even if you're young enough that you don't care that much about aging now, you will someday—and it will come along sooner than you think.

As a California native, I grew up believing that pasty white legs were to be avoided at all costs. Spring break wasn't really spring break unless you went someplace (even if it was just someone's backyard) where you bobbed on a noodle in an outdoor pool, played lots and lots of beer pong, and came back a warm golden bronze. We thought that a good tan looked happy and healthy and was synonymous with the relaxing joys of being on vacation.

At the same time, my L.A. County hometown had a pretty big Asian immigrant population, so it was a common sight to see Korean moms driving in their minivans while wearing a full face visor, gloves, and fake sleeves that went up to the armpits—all to protect their skin from the sun. From the outside looking in, it might seem a little bit cray cray to take sun care that seriously. I know it did to my friends and me, and we cracked more than a few jokes at our moms' expense.

A straddler in both worlds, I avoided anything that might resemble this crazy, overprotective route. All that changed when I went to Korea and saw first-hand that it wasn't just nerdy older ladies who were conscious about sun exposure. In Seoul, protecting your skin from the sun was smart and savvy and something that everybody did.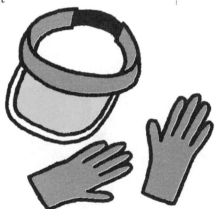

So I bought some sunscreen, and sometimes I even remembered to wear it. But I'd still skimp on cloudy days, or when I knew I was going to be inside most of the time, and didn't take my sun protection all that seriously. What really drove it home and made me a believer was when I started my esthetician training and began to study the science behind skin.

Sunscreen is the real deal. Not to be dramatic, but it can keep you looking years younger *and,* when it comes to skin cancer, save your life. Still, though, I've met tons of people who don't think twice about going out of their way to eat organic, or spend money on expensive yoga lessons for their well-being, yet let sun protection fall low on their list of priorities. For some reason, a lot of us still tend to think of sunscreen as a negotiable part of our beauty routine, and this couldn't be further from the truth.

There's a Korean proverb that goes "Where you plant a soybean, you will get a soybean. Where you plant a red bean, you will get a red bean." Did I lose you? Ha, well, this is just a long-winded way of saying you reap what you sow. And if you neglect your sun care, twenty to thirty years down the line you'll regret that you didn't plant a few dozen acres of soybeans and red beans. Your regret might even be written right across your face—in the form of age spots, wrinkles, and sagging skin.

Sun Protection Myths and Facts

While Western popular consciousness is no doubt catching up, Koreans have been in this "stay out of the sun" game for way longer. While I was in Southern California, slathering on suntan lotion to turn my skin a deeper shade of brown, my Korean counterparts halfway around the world were dodging direct sunlight at all costs. When I got to Seoul, I was surprised to see that even on particularly sunny, beautiful days, I'd see many people forgoing a view of the clear blue sky in favor of the protection of sun umbrellas. In California, this didn't happen—people moved there specifically for the sun.

Sure, the sun feels great on your shoulders, and we've been conditioned to believe that we look better with a tan. Still, the sun is not our friend, and there's actually no such thing as a "healthy" glow because it can actually damage the skin, increase your risk of cancer, and age your skin prematurely. So how do we change our mindset and start taking our sun protection as seriously as we should? Well, first we have to be convinced that it's actually worth our time. To do that, I want to address some common questions and misgivings that you might have about protecting yourself from the sun.

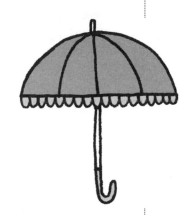

I hear about UVA and UVB all the time and see it on sunscreen labels. What's the difference?

You're not alone if you are confused about what the different numbers and acronyms stand for on a standard sunscreen product. UV stands for "ultraviolet radiation," which is a form of energy that comes from the sun. UV spells disaster for your skin, and it's been deemed a *human carcinogen* (the term given to any substance or radiation that is cancer causing) because it causes damage to the skin's cellular DNA.

- The *A* in UVA stands for aging ray and has a long wavelength, which means it penetrates deep into the skin (the dermis). It's not only a cancer creator, but it plays a major role in aging because it attacks the collagen in your dermis. You should hate it.

- *B* stands for burning and has a shorter wavelength than the UVA ray, so it penetrates the skin more superficially. UVB is the main cause of skin cancers, and you can also thank it for that sunburn you got last summer. You should hate it, too.

It's best to use a sunscreen that contains both UVA and UVB protection. Look for a sunscreen labeled "broad spectrum protection," which means it has passed the critical wavelength test to protect from both aging and burning rays. See the chart below to see what ingredients protect against which specific rays.

Chemical Absorbers	Protects Against
Aminobenzoic Acid (PABA)	UVB
Avobenzone	UVA1
Cinoxate	UVB
Dioxybenzone	UVB, UVA2
Ecamsule (Mexoryl SX)	UVA2
Ensulizole (Phenylbenzimidazole Sulfonic Acid)	UVB
Homosalate	UVB
Meradimate (Menthyl Anthranilate)	UVA2
Octinoxate (Octyl Methoxycinnamate)	UVB
Octisalate (Octyl Salicylate)	UVB
Octocrylene	UVB
Oxybenzone	UVB, UVA2

Chemical Absorbers	Protects Against
Padimate O	UVB
Sulisobenzone	UVB, UVA2
Trolamine Salicylate	UVB
Physical Filters	
Titanium Dioxide	UVB, UVA2
Zinc Oxide	UVB, UVA2, UVA1
Source: skincancer.org	

FYI, the FDA no longer allows companies to label their products as "sunblock," because no lotion can block the sun completely; it can only screen out some of the UV rays. Hence the term *sunscreen*.

So what does UV do to my skin?

You'll be amazed to know how much UV rays actually act like laser beams, shooting into your dermis and damaging collagen fibers (proteins that give structure to the skin) and elastin (a protein that creates the spring in the tissue beneath the skin). Also, some of the damage is collateral damage. When your elastin starts breaking down, the body produces enzymes called metalloproteinases (also referred to as

MMP), which further contribute to collagen breakdown and even more wrinkles.

Similarly, when the UV rays damage the cellular DNA of your skin, your body tries to fix the DNA, a process that itself produces toxic free radicals. These unstable free radicals destroy everything in their path, causing wrinkles, sunspots, and skin cancers. Products and foods that are labeled or called "antioxidant" help fight free radicals.

Now I'm scared of free radicals and UV. What do I do?

Wear your sunscreen.

There are two main types of sunscreen that keep the evil rays away from the cellular DNA and collagen in the dermis.

Physical sunscreen (also known as mineral sunscreen) sits on the skin like armor and forms a barrier between the sun and your skin to keep rays from penetrating. Titanium dioxide and zinc oxide are classic mineral sunscreen ingredients. Remember back in the day when lifeguards had that patch of white on their noses? That was mineral sunscreen, so it's been around for a long time. The plus side of mineral-based sunscreens is that they're gentle on the skin (and won't irritate conditions like rosacea, which can be supersensitive to both the sun and sunscreen) and they work immediately upon application. With technological advances such as nanotechnology, many sunscreens are now formulated to be lightweight, blendable, and nongreasy, so your nose won't look like a lifeguard's.

A chemical sunscreen (also known as synthetic sunscreen) filters the radiation by absorbing it and then transforming it into heat energy. Because it's a chemical process, you should give it about fifteen minutes after application for it to soak in and work effectively.

Chemical sunscreens can be a lot lighter than mineral formulas, and most go on like moisturizers, leaving no visible traces. Chemical sunscreens typically contain a combination of two to six active ingredients, such as oxybenzone, avobenzone, or octisalate. Some environmental groups claim that chemical sunscreens (as well as some physical ones) can absorb into the skin and bloodstream, causing everything from allergic reactions to hormone disruptions. There are also other groups (including the FDA) that have published studies claiming that chemical sunscreens do not have harmful side effects and can be used on children six months and older.

There are many sides to this story, but my two cents is that you will be healthier and safer overall if you use sunscreen than if you do not use it at all. If you're truly concerned, I'd recommend zinc oxide or titanium oxide sunscreens that do not have nanoparticle-size ingredients and therefore cannot be absorbed into your bloodstream.

What does SPF mean, and how do I pick a number?

First things first: SPF stands for "sun protection factor," and it measures how effective the sunscreen is at blocking UVB rays. There are different models for measuring SPF. One is based on time: If it takes ten minutes of direct sun exposure for your unprotected skin to turn red, putting on SPF 15 will give you approximately 2.5 hours of sun protection (SPF 15 x 10 minutes = 150 minutes). Most people start to burn within five to ten minutes, but those with fair skin can start to sizzle almost immediately, especially in direct sunlight. Another is based on the strength of the formula: SPF 15 blocks 93 to 95 percent of UVB rays; SPF 30 blocks 97 percent of UVB rays; SPF 50 blocks 98 percent of UVB rays; and so on and so forth. Neither of these models is perfect, but both can give you some sense of the difference between SPFs and how that impacts your level of sun exposure. Your skin burning and turning red is an indication of damage from UVB rays, but you can still sustain a lot of UVA damage without these warning signs, so don't assume you're in the safe zone just because you don't see any signs of sunburn.

As you can see, despite the jump in sun protection factor from the number 15 to 50, there's a plateau in the amount of protection that you're getting. That's why the FDA created tighter regulations around SPF labeling. You can no longer buy products that say SPF 100, and companies now must label anything over SPF 50 as 50+.

So if I'm wearing waterproof SPF 50, I'm good all day, right?

Wrong. Pay no heed to any "waterproof" or "sweat-proof" claims on products. In fact, the FDA no longer allows companies to market sunscreens with these words, because they're simply misleading.

If you're sweating or swimming, your sunscreen will undoubtedly wash off and you won't be as protected as you were. The common rule of thumb is that you should reapply your sunscreen every two to three hours. If you're sweating, reapply even more often than that. Swimming? It's a good idea to reapply every time you come out of the water.

> *I'm good at math. If I combine my SPF 15 moisturizer with my SPF 30 BB cream, does that equal SPF 45?*

Nope. When you combine two products with different SPFs, your total sun protection factor will be equivalent to the highest SPF you applied—in this case, 30. But don't let this stop you from layering. Protection is protection, and the more products you use with an SPF, the better.

> *I've seen a lot of brands with a "PA" and the + symbol. What do they stand for?*

PA is actually a rating developed in Japan to determine the amount of UVA protection a product offers, in addition to the standard way SPF measures UVB protection. Japanese researchers developed the PA system by converting the existing PPD (persistent pigment darkening) rating system, which measures skin-aging UVA rays. You will see ratings like PA+ Low UVA protection, PA++ Moderate UVA protection, or PA+++ High UVA protection.

> *You're preaching to the choir—I wear sunscreen when I go to the beach or Coachella.*

Bravo! That's a *start*! Now how about incorporating sunscreen as part of your daily routine? In fact, most of our sun exposure doesn't come from the beach or entire days outside, but from everyday exposure that adds up over time.

Even on a ten-minute walk around the block with your pup, your face is being attacked and damaged by the sun's rays. Also, don't let an overcast day fool you. The majority of UVA and UVB rays can still penetrate clouds. Even on a snowy day, 80 percent of the rays can reflect off the snow directly onto you.

If you're inside but near a window, you're getting sun exposure. If you're riding in a car, damaging rays still come through the window. If you've got a flight during the day and you plan to have your window shade up, put on that sunscreen! The sun is even more damaging at higher altitudes, so think about that when you're getting on a plane, or hanging out in Denver.

> *Whatever, Charlotte—you're Asian, so of course you have good skin. Skin is all genetics.*

You're partly right, but not totally. You do inherit your skin type from your parents, but your genes account for only 10 to 20 percent of aging. A mind-blowing 80 to 90 percent of your aging is a result of environmental factors.

In 2012, truck driver Bill McElligott's sun damage made international news. At sixty-nine years old, McElligott had driven a truck for twenty-eight years without wearing sunscreen, leaving the left side of his face exposed to the sun through the driver's side window. The difference between the left side of his face and the right, which was shaded and got significantly less exposure, was shocking. The left side was saggy, wrinkly, and spotty and looked twenty years older than the right. It looked like special effects out of a movie—Google his name and you can see this cautionary tale for real.

While McElligott's case was extreme, he's not alone, and most people in the United States who drive a lot have more sun damage on the left sides of their faces. In the United Kingdom, where drivers sit on the right side, it's reversed, with the right sides of their faces aged significantly more than the left. So think about that the next time you jump in the car and head to Target.

> *Fine. I'll wear sunscreen. If I wear SPF 50, can I call it a day?*

Oh, if only life were that simple! Even if you put sunscreen on in the morning, you'll still need to reapply throughout the day. Reapplication is key because SPF protection fades and is ineffective after a few hours' time—even if you haven't sweat a single drop. If you're spending most of your day inside, out of the sun, this is where cushion compacts and makeup with sunscreen really come in handy, because you won't have to completely start over to reapply. You can just freshen up your makeup and your SPF at the same time.

#SoKoSecret: One of the one million reasons to love cushion compacts is that most have SPF and are formulated to be applied over and over again throughout the day. You can touch up your makeup and reapply your SPF in one go.

But seriously, I just hate wearing sunscreen.

If you haven't tried it lately, you're probably not aware of the huge improvements in products with SPF. Nowadays, there are a lot of lightweight, nongreasy, nonpasty-looking sunscreen options, so keep trying new ones until you find one that you like (a lot of Korean beauty companies are really generous with samples, but sadly, a lot of U.S. companies are still lagging behind in this department).

Also, the less you like wearing sunscreen, the more reason to splurge on those sunglasses and hats. Make sure you go for lenses with 100 percent UVA and UVB absorption (and the bigger the frames, the better) and that your hats have a decent brim that actually shades your face.

I personally don't leave the house in the daytime without sunglasses, because they protect the skin around my eyes, which is the thinnest and most delicate and needs all the protection it can get. Now, when I'm working as an esthetician and giving treatments, I really notice the sun damage that people have under and around their eyes.

Also, some clothing (such as a long-sleeved cotton T-shirt) will protect you, but only at a very low level, the equivalent of around an SPF 5.

Am I good if I use SPF makeup?

SPF makeup is a start, but you're probably not applying nearly the amount of product necessary to get the protection you need. SPF makeup often gives you a false sense of sun-protection security, because you can't rely on it alone to do the job.

When companies make claims about SPF protection, they're usually testing a tablespoon of product. If you're not using that much, then the level of sun protection you're getting is far less than what it says on the bottle. So don't skimp on your sunscreen—it'll pay off.

But I really need a tan! I'm so pasty!

Been there, done that, so I completely understand where you're coming from. Especially if you're on a vacation, a tan is the most envy-inducing souvenir you can bring back. I'm sorry to break it to you, but do you want to know what a tan really is? Visible sun damage. So, how do you like them coconuts?

When UV rays attack your skin, your body tries to protect itself from the damage by producing melanin, the pigment that causes your skin to tan. Unfortunately this whole process causes cell mutations and produces free radicals.

Also, forgo the tanning beds. Those should have stayed back in the 1980s where they belong. There's a reason they're shaped like coffins— they damage your skin and can cause skin cancers.

#SoKoSecret: Have you ever noticed when someone's skin has a lot of white spots? That's sun damage, too—those cells have been so tapped out that they literally can no longer produce melanin. It's kind of sad. Poor cells.

You only need sunscreen when you're older.

Actually, sunscreen is even more crucial before age eighteen, because a whopping 80 percent of your total lifetime sun exposure takes place before you exit high school. That's right—you accumulate major UVA damage from those teenage tans, and it's a huge factor in the pigmentation that you'll start to see come out on your face decades later.

Parents in Korea are extra vigilant, and you often see them slathering their kids with sunscreen, shielding them with wide-brimmed hats, and urging them to stay in the shade. This helps make sun protection a habit kids grow up with, so it's not just another chore to add to their routine as an adult.

For me, I can't change the fact that I refused to wear sunscreen during the long hours I spent outside as a cheerleader, passionately cheering on the flag football team as the cocaptain of the junior high squad. But I do know I'll make my kids, nephews, and nieces (and any child within shouting distance) grow up with this knowledge, and a good bottle of sunscreen.

#SoKoSecret: Mineral sunscreens are great for kids. Formulated with zinc or titanium oxide, they're less likely to irritate sensitive skin.

I guess it's too late for me, then.

Not at all. You'll reap the benefits from being sun savvy at any age, especially when it comes to protecting yourself from skin cancer! According to the American Cancer Society, skin cancer is the most common cancer, accounting for nearly half of cancers in the United States. But in sun-vigilant Korea, skin cancer doesn't even make the list of the ten most common cancers! Coincidence? Methinks not.

If you have a family history of skin cancer, you should be extra careful. Watch out for any sores that don't heal, moles that change size or color, or spots on your skin that feel extra tender or painful.

> *Fine. I'll wear sunscreen. What else do I need to know about it?*

Don't forget to apply sunscreen to your lips, hands, chest, ears, neck, and shoulders. You ever wonder why these areas are the most telltale signs of a person's age? Because they're often neglected in the skin-care process and also pretty consistently exposed to the sun. You should use a nickel-size amount of sunscreen for your face and an equal amount for your neck and chest.

Also, as I mentioned in chapter five, you need to be extra cautious about sun protection after you exfoliate or use products that contain retinol.

Sunscreen should be the last part of your skin-care routine, because applying anything on top of it (like a moisturizer) will dilute it. Wait at least four minutes after putting on your SPF to apply makeup, and make sure your makeup includes SPF as well. See page 113 for some of my favorite sunscreens.

SKIN STORIES: Dave Cho

SOKO GLAM COFOUNDER (AND MY HUSBAND)

I have to give my mom some major props. I remember when I was a young, overweight elementary school kid (with Coke-bottle glasses *and* braces), my mom taught me to always, always wear sunscreen and to use facial soap, not bar soap, for my face. Skin care is all about prevention and being proactive, so I'm thankful that I was educated at such a young age.

Before Soko Glam, I spent more than eight years on active duty in the U.S. Army as a combat arms officer, serving almost the entire time overseas (including a deployment to the Middle East). I've experienced extreme weather conditions (over 130°F in the desert and −30°F in the Arctic tundra) and gone weeks without clean, running water. To say the least, my skin has taken quite a beating. But even through all of this, I still get compliments on my skin, and people ask what kind of products I use for my face. Maybe it's because while others were sleeping or eating chow, I took a quick few minutes to do what was necessary: apply SPF. Most of the time, the questions come from women, but sometimes (discreetly) from men as well.

I wear SPF on my face every single day without fail. Recently, I had unexplained pain and required a trip to the emergency room, but I still took the time to put on sunscreen before I left the house somehow—it sounds crazy, but it's more like muscle memory now. Whenever Charlotte checks out my skin under a Wood's lamp (a black light that reveals the condition of the skin under the surface), she sees very little pigmentation. This is probably because I've religiously worn sunscreen ever since I was a kid. So again, thanks, Mom!

The KoRean 10 step Skin-care RoUTiNE*

① Makeup Remover and OIL CLEANSER
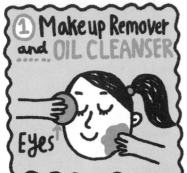
Eyes

♡② WATER-BASED cleanser
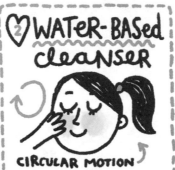
CIRCULAR MOTION

③ ExFoliaToR
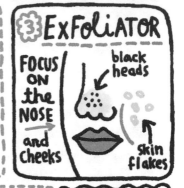
FOCUS ON the NOSE and cheeks
black heads
skin flakes

✿④ TONER
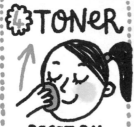
RESET P.H. and HYDRATE!

⑤ Essence
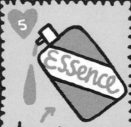
to NOURISH and renew

⑥ AMPOULES
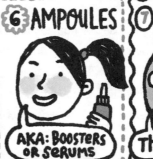
AKA: BOOSTERS OR SERUMS

⑦ SHEET mask
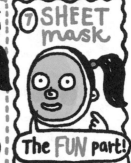
The FUN part!

⑧ Eye CREAM
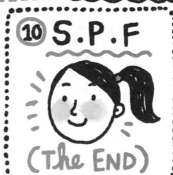
GENTLY TAP WITH YOUR PINKY FINGER

✿⑨ MoistuRizeR
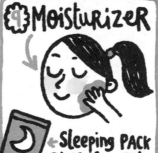
Sleeping PACK once A week

⑩ S.P.F
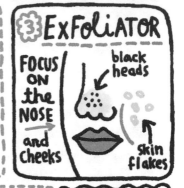
(The END)

* NOTE : Not all steps need to be done on a daily basis!

The Mysterious Ten-Step Korean Skin-Care Routine—

Demystified!

*I*f you're familiar with any aspect of Korean beauty, it's probably the *famous ten-step Korean skin-care routine!!!* It's gotten a ton of press over the last few years, and it's easy to see why: It's a bit shocking. *Geez Louise,* you think, *ten steps is a lot. Those Korean women sure are high maintenance . . .*

But here's the thing: While Korean women do typically include more products in their skin-care routine than their American counterparts, it's not as if they're using all ten products twice a day every day. Whether it's daily, every other day, or weekly, each product enters the rotation for a specific purpose. Some you might even use only once a month, or only during a certain season.

When I first started going over to my friends' houses in Seoul, my eyes would bulge when I saw the stacks of products above their sinks. But as they would patiently explain what each product was for, I started to see the point. "This is for my T-zone, because I get an oily shine early in the day," a friend would say as she gave me a guided tour of her vanity. "This treats the brown spots along my cheeks, and these are the moisturizers I use in the summer." I had always believed in a quality-over-quantity and less-is-more philosophy, but I could tell she knew what she was talking about. Besides, her skin was gorgeous, so she was definitely doing something right.

Treat Your Skin with the Respect That It Deserves

I'm a big believer that there is only one person who will motivate you to do things that require discipline: you. But if you're hearing about the ten steps and thinking, *No way, not me. I barely have time to shave my pits and trim my toenails,* I get it, because that's what I thought at first, too. But whatever you may hear, there are no miracle cures, and the only true way to get good skin is to invest a little time and effort.

Many of us have started a skin-care routine out of fear (*Oh my God, I'm going to look like my mother!*) or to reverse damage we've already done (*These brown spots weren't here last month!*). Or if you're like me, sometimes all it takes is a semipublic shaming from some well-meaning coworkers. All of these work, but the best and most lasting motivation is the desire to treat your skin-care routine as part of your overall well-being.

When you're a busy person, it's easy to forget about your skin. Because let's be honest, you can always cover it up (at least temporarily). With the right angles, filters, makeup, and lighting, good skin can easily be faked. But you can't spend your entire life by candlelight, and reality doesn't come with Photoshop. And when you're young, you think you and your skin are invincible. "Your UV rays don't hurt me!" you say while shaking your fist at the sun. Then one day you blink and wake up to brown spots, fine lines, congested pores, and borderline eczema. But before you get depressed and go lie down on the couch (out of the sun), let me assure you: These skin-care woes are avoidable. Adopting your own arsenal of steps (whether it's four or ten) is one of the first lines of defense.

When you start to think about putting together your own skin-care routine, don't be intimidated by the idea that you'll have to spend a certain amount of money, use only Korean products, or buy products you don't need. Every Korean woman's skin-care routine is different, because every skin has different needs. This information is just a guideline to show the order of the steps and give you a sense of the products that you can use regularly.

Good skin is not about having more products than you can count—it's about having the right products that do the right things and then using them in the right order. You need to properly cleanse, exfoliate, treat, moisturize, and protect your skin, and believe it or not, all of this should take only five to ten minutes in the morning and another five to ten at night. If you're like me—a night owl—then you'll probably want to perform the steps that you don't do every day (like exfoliation and masks) at night when you have the time to unwind. If the morning is when you have extra time and energy to devote to your skin-care routine, then by all means, grab your OJ and go for it (I share my morning routine on page 114).

Now, read on, you low-maintenance lady—this routine's for you, too.

The Korean Ten-Step Skin-Care Routine

1. Makeup Remover and Oil Cleanser

On days when I wear a lot of makeup (especially waterproof mascara and a lip stain), I start my routine with a cotton pad soaked in gentle makeup remover or an oil-based cleansing tissue. This helps remove eye makeup precisely, which may not seem like a big deal, but you want to get all your mascara off, as your eyes and eyelashes are delicate enough as it is without being caked with a week's worth of old mascara.

After that, I use an oil cleanser on the rest of my face. Apply on dry face directly with your fingers, and use gentle, upward circular motions. Contrary to popular belief, even those with oily skin can use an oil cleanser—it won't make you oilier. What it will do is break down all the oil-based debris that's left on your skin, such as makeup, sunscreen, and sebum, as well as smog and pollution.

My picks:

3 Concept Eyes Lip & Eye Remover gently eliminates all traces of waterproof mascaras, eyeliners, and lip stains.

Banila Co. Clean It Zero Classic is a sorbet-soft, lightweight formula that transforms from a solid balm to a silky oil on the skin and effortlessly dissolves stubborn makeup and dirt.

Tony Moly Floria Brightening Cleansing Oil gently whisks away makeup and washes away sebum and brightens the skin tone with the superstar fermented ingredient saccharomyces ferment.

Skinfood Brown Rice Oil Cleansing Tissue comes with forty premoistened wipes containing vitamins and antioxidants from rice bran.

2. Water-Based Cleanser

Now it's time to wash your face again, and no, I'm not kidding. Cleansing twice is not only practiced by Koreans, but it's actually recommended by many estheticians and dermatologists because it helps to thoroughly remove any impurities that can cause breakouts. Apply a water-based cleanser, which will usually be creamy in texture or foam up when you add water, to a wet face, and work it in circular motions with your fingers. During both cleanses, gently massage the face to help increase circulation and enhance lymphatic drainage.

My picks:

Neogen Dermalogy Real Fresh Green Tea Foam is a light cleanser formulated for sensitive skin types, is made with green tea extract to fight free radicals, and leaves skin feeling soft and moisturized.

Su:m37 Miracle Rose Cleansing Stick has convenient twist-as-you-go tube packaging that works into a gentle lather. It's made with fermented damask rose extract and rose petals.

Benton Honest Cleansing Foam begins as a rich cream, and transforms into a luxurious foam. Leaves skin soft and moisturized with botanical extracts.

3. The Exfoliator

Don't underestimate the importance of exfoliating! It helps loosen debris in clogged pores and sloughs off dead skin cells, which can improve your skin's texture, brighten your complexion, and help your other products absorb better. You can use a mechanical exfoliator, like a sugar scrub, or a chemical one, which uses ingredients like lactic or salicylic acid to dissolve the "glue" that binds dead skin cells to healthy ones. Exfoliate once or twice a week, and focus on your nose (where blackheads love to party) and the visible pores on your cheeks. Don't forget to lightly scrub your lips, too, which keeps them soft and helps your lipstick go on smoothly.

My picks:

Skinfood Black Sugar Mask Wash Off is a nourishing wash-off mask that promotes hydration and the sloughing of dead skin cells for better product absorption.

Neogen Bio-Peel Gauze Peeling Wine uses physical exfoliating pads soaked in tartaric acid (AHA) to chemically exfoliate and to promote clearer, smoother, and tighter skin.

AmorePacific Treatment Enzyme Peel uses natural papaya enzymes to eliminate dry, dull surface cells for a smoother and brighter complexion.

Goodal Phytowash Yerba Mate Bubble Peeling is an innovative "peeling" exfoliator that transforms from a creamy serum into a foamy exfoliator to gently remove dead skin cells.

4. The Toner

Toner is an in-between step and often the step people will tell you to skip if you're trying to simplify your skin-care routine. But don't listen to the naysayers! Toners are actually very important. Used after cleansing, they help remove any leftover residues from your cleanser while also prepping and repairing your skin's barrier to effectively absorb the moisturizers that follow.

In Korea, a lot of women use hydrating toners instead of astringent ones, and you can find ones that are suitable for all skin types. They're packed with humectants that aid in soothing and hydrating, which is why toners are often called "refreshers" by Korean brands. Use a cotton pad to swipe it all across your face and neck or you can pat in the product with your hands.

#SoKoSecret Chances are it'll be hard to find a Korean toner that uses witch hazel or some sort of alcohol; consumers generally stay away from products with alcohol because it dries out the skin!

My picks:

RE:P Organic Cotton Treatment Toning Pad balances and soothes the skin with chamomile and lavender. The organic cotton pad offers gentle exfoliation to remove impurities.

Son & Park Beauty Water is a smart cleansing liquid made from natural plant extracts that tones, exfoliates and hydrates to deliver smooth and revitalized skin.

Su:m37 Water-full Skin Refresher hydrates and balances the skin with ingredients such as bamboo water and red clover flower.

Missha Time Revolution Clear Toner is a fragrance-free highly enriched hydrating toner formulated with fermented ingredients that helps even out the skin tone and preps the skin to absorb the rest of the skin-care routine.

5. The Essence

Aw, the essence—the heart of the Korean skin-care routine! Korean women consider essence the most important step; it's a skin-care category that was created in Korea. Essence is still hard to find elsewhere, but I bet that won't be the case much longer! I've also had the most noticeable results from adding this to my regimen, because essences help hydrate and increase cell turnover. Hello, brighter skin!

#SoKoSecret. A lot of Korean women also use an essence on their hair as well. A hair essence helps make your strands shinier and softer and provides brittle hair with nutrients. Whenever I would get my hair done in Seoul, my stylist would also give me a stern scolding when I'd cop to using an essence only every once in a while instead of every time I washed my hair.

My picks:

Missha Time Revolution First Treatment Essence improves elasticity and evens out skin tone by promoting skin renewal with its superstar ingredient, saccharomyces ferment filtrate.

Neogen Code 9 Lemon Green Caviar Essence & Tox Tightening Pack uses a unique triple-layer sheet pad soaked in cell-communicating ingredients to even out skin tone and deliver nutrients to the skin.

IOPE Bio Essence Intensive Conditioning has more than eighty fermented ingredients that promote clear, healthy, hydrated skin.

6. Ampoules, Boosters, and Serums

Ampoules, which are often referred to as serums and boosters in Western lines, are what you would get if you put an essence on the stove and boiled it down until it was just the good stuff. They usually have a thicker consistency and are used to target and treat very specific skin problems. They can help brighten skin (by increasing cell turnover, as I've said before), fade sunspots, and smooth fine lines.

My picks:

Klairs Freshly Juiced Vitamin C Drop Serum revitalizes the skin by brightening and reducing the visibility of dark spots and acne scars.

Missha Time Revolution Night Repair New Science Activator Ampoule is a mouthful, but is awesome as a spot treatment to reduce signs of aging, improve skin elasticity, and protect barrier function.

RE:P Ultra Moist Gel Oil an advanced serum that intensively replenishes rough, dry skin with argan and jojoba seed oils.

7. The Sheet Mask

If the essence is the heart of the Korean skin-care routine, then the sheet mask is the soul. It's the quiet, meditative ritual of relaxation. On average, you should use a sheet mask twice a week, but you can do it more often if your face is very dry. The fun of sheet masks is in the variety and the price—sometimes you can even grab one for a dollar.

Place a sheet mask on your face and then lie back and chill out for twenty minutes. The secret to sheet masks is that the sheet helps keep the product from evaporating, and its prolonged contact with your face forces your skin to absorb more of the nutrients and moisture than if you just applied them via a cream or serum.

My picks:

Manefit Bling Bling Hydrogel Mask is a two-piece mask soaked in nourishing essences that instantly cools and soothes stressed, tired skin on contact.

Tony Moly My Little Pet Eye Patch uses green tea extract and niacinamide to revitalize, moisturize, and reduce the visibility of fine lines and dull under-eye skin.

Skinfood Hydro Fitting Snail Mask Sheet uses snail mucin to encourage cell regeneration, soothe irritated skin, and replenish moisture levels.

Banila Co It Radiant Lace Hydrogel Mask Sheet hydrates and nourishes the skin with ingredients such as aloe. The clear and white lace pattern makes sheet masking chic.

8. The Eye Cream

If the eyes are the windows to your soul, then the skin around them is the barometer of your age (just doesn't sound as poetic, does it?). Regularly using an intensive eye cream can help keep dark circles, puffiness, and crow's-feet at bay. The skin around your eyes is the thinnest and most delicate skin on your face, and eye creams are similar to ampoules and essences, but packed with a higher concentration of beneficial ingredients and formulated to be extra gentle and nonirritating.

To apply eye cream, you want to use your pinkie to gently tap the product around the entire orbital bone, and don't get too close to the waterlines of your eyes or you can irritate them. We've all seen sleepy children rub their eyes, so think of that as the exact opposite of what you want to do here. Not only does tapping your eye cream on lead to better absorption of the product, but it also eliminates the tugging and pulling that just cause more wrinkles!

My picks:

Skinfood Royal Honey Eye Cream is made with hydrating humectants such as royal jelly and honey extract and comes in a hygienic tube.

Banila Co It Radiant Brightening Eye Cream uses natural ingredients to hydrate and soothe stressed and delicate skin.

Etude House Moistfull Super Collagen Eye Concentrate is made with a unique baobab seed oil formula that smooths out fine lines and wrinkles.

9. The Moisturizer

Hydration is probably the most important part of your nighttime skin-care routine (sorry, moisturizing, but sunscreen is the most important part of your day routine—more on that later). It's likely the thickest formula that you'll apply to your face, which is why it goes on last, and it will make the most out of your skin's restorative midnight hours. Once a week, sub in a sleeping pack in place of your night cream to (surprise, surprise) hydrate intensely.

My picks:

Son & Park Beauty Gel is a moisturizing gel that cools the skin and creates a dewy, fresh glow. Perfect before makeup application.

LIZ K Ultra Waterfall Cream is a gel-based moisturizer that intensely hydrates, brightens, and soothes throughout the day and night.

Goodal Super Seed Oil Plus Balancing Emulsion uses fermented seed oils to improve skin elasticity, even skin tone, decrease redness, and inhibit excess oil production.

Missha Super Aqua Cell Renew Snail Cream is a gel cream with snail mucin (an extract with skin-beneficial ingredients such as hyaluronic acid and glycoprotein enzymes), which restores hydration and repairs damaged skin.

Belif True Cream—Aqua Bomb is a light gel cream formulated to "burst" when applied to deliver extra hydration and moisture to the skin for a healthy, supple complexion.

Lioele V-Line Waterdrop Sleeping Pack also has a gel consistency, is deeply hydrating, and reduces redness. Massage the formula into the skin and it transforms into water droplets.

RE:P All Night Moisture And Relief Mask is a sleeping mask infused with botanical extracts from lemon, basil, and olive to restore and renew the skin.

10. Sunscreen

The final product here could also count as steps 11, 12, and 13, since you'll be reapplying throughout the day. Regularly wearing SPF, even if you're just sitting near a window or stepping outside for a few minutes, is probably the number one thing you can do to maintain and protect the health and beauty of your skin.

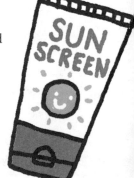

#SoKoSecret: It's super important to use sunscreen after exfoliation or any laser treatments! Your skin is more fragile after those procedures. Breakouts are also technically small wounds and are therefore more susceptible to post-inflammatory pigmentation, which is why sometimes after a pimple heals a brown spot takes its place.

My picks:

Skinfood Gold Kiwi Sun Cream is a lightweight, nongreasy broad spectrum SPF 50+/PA+++ that also uses zinc oxide and titanium dioxide to protect the skin from UVA/UVB damage.

Neogen Day-Light Protection Sun Screen SPF 50/PA+++ offers broad spectrum protection for sensitive skin types.

Missha All-Around Safe Block Waterproof Sun Milk is a light facial sunscreen that absorbs quickly, without a greasy or white cast, and protects skin with zinc oxide and titanium dioxide for SPF 50+/PA+++ broad spectrum protection.

In Skin Care, as in Life, Change Is Good

Even once you've established a skin-care routine, it's still not set in stone. You might want to add or subtract products when the seasons change (such as using an additional moisturizing cream in the winter, or switching to a lighter emulsion in the summer), or when you're traveling between dif-

The Ten-Step Routine

ferent climates. That's why it's so important to get to know your skin and what works for you. No skin-care routine is one-size-fits-all, nor is there a guarantee that what gives you great results now will work just as well a year from now.

Tweaking Your Routine for Morning (Or, How to Get to Work on Time)

My day routine is similar to my night routine, but since I'm usually in a frantic rush to make up for hitting snooze on my alarm a few times, I usually work with just the essentials.

I start with a double cleanse. Even in the morning? Yes! You just spent (hopefully) six to eight hours sleeping with your skin-care products on, all while sweating and producing oil. Trust me—you're going to want to wash that off with the double cleanse. Then I follow with a toner, just as at night, then my hydrating routine of essence, ampoule, or serum (depending on what I'm using at that particular time), eye cream, and moisturizer.

After I've given those products time to absorb (usually while I brush my teeth, brush my hair, slurp a smoothie), I finish off with a generous layer of sunscreen, and then move on to my makeup.

Sometimes, you might skip one of your cleansing or moisturizing steps in the morning—and of course it won't kill you. But sunscreen is the absolute essential component of the day routine if you're going to get even five minutes of sun exposure. It's possible that your day moisturizer, BB cream, or cushion compact has SPF, but just make sure that you're getting adequate sun protection.

#SoKoSecret: As much as the multi-step, layering approach is popular in Korea, beauty brands are starting to come out with single formulas that both tone and exfoliates in one go. The latest buzz worthy product is *Son & Park's* Beauty Water, which has extracts of orange, lavender, and rose.

SKIN STORIES: Yeon-seo Oh

SOUTH KOREAN ACTRESS AND MODEL

First I wash my face with a mild oil cleanser and rinse, and then I massage with a soft cleansing foam, then rinse thoroughly with water. My favorite item is Neogen Dermalogy Real Fresh Foam because it has natural fruits and gives you a clear baby face.

I follow with toner and moisturize right away with essence. I don't like creams that are too rich or have a heavy texture, so I always use Neogen Tox Tightening Pack before going to sleep. I know that when I massage and hydrate my skin at night, my makeup will look better the next day. I'm always working with makeup artists, and I get a lot of tips from them. They touch and care for my skin almost every day, so they tell me which products are good and how to use them. I feel like that has really helped me learn how to care for my skin.

I wear makeup as part of my job, but skin care is the most important and should come before everything. If you have healthy and glowing skin, then you just need a little touch of makeup.

What's YOUR skin type?

NORMAL

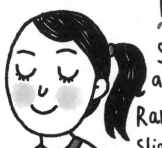

Some pores along T-zone.
Rare breakouts.
Slight oily shine.

DRY

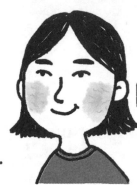

Little to no pores or shine.
Flaky & tight skin.

OILY

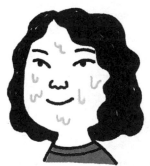

Frequent breakouts.
Large pores.
Oily shine.

COMBINATION

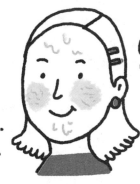

Oily T-zone, dry elsewhere.

SENSITIVE

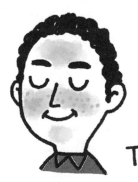

Skin reacts easily to products / environment.
Turns red, bumpy or itchy.

The ABCs of Skin-Care Shopping:

Finding the Right Products for You

Now that you're thoroughly pumped to start your skin-care routine, where do you start? You start shopping.

But before you go all Cher Horowitz on beauty products, be warned: Shopping for skin care can often feel overwhelming because of the choices and the prices. Do you need an essence, a sleeping pack, or a sheet mask? Wait, do you need all three? Should your oil cleanser come with a pump or in balm form? Oh my God, you forgot about eye cream!

Or it can be underwhelming if you're expecting your skin to improve, but end up with a product that causes more congestion on your face than you started with—a one-way ticket to bummer city.

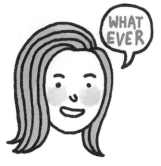

So instead of grabbing your credit card and heading out blind, let's do some soul searching and assess the best way to go about purchasing skin-care products for you. I'm also a firm believer that you can respect your skin and your wallet at the same time, so let's make smart choices here, people!

First things first: Refresher course! Remember when I told you that you shouldn't just assume that what your two best friends are using will suit you? No matter how much they rave about a product, it just might not be right for you. Your skin is uniquely yours.

After speaking with dermatologists in Korea and R&D specialists of top Korean beauty companies and pairing their info with my own esthetician knowledge, I put together some guidelines on what conditions you might see on your face and how to use that information to help determine *your* skin type. I stress the word "guideline" because obviously there's no perfect formula and your skin's conditions can change depending on several different factors. Environmental conditions, stress levels, allergies, and diet are just some of the things that play a role in your skin condition and keep it constantly changing.

This is why my time in front of the mirror is not limited to applying makeup or trying on different shoes. I take time to really analyze my skin and see how it's doing. Don't be afraid to get up close and personal with the mirror after you cleanse your face. Take the time to really look at your skin using not only your eyes, but your fingers, too, as they can feel things your eyes may not be able to catch! Once a week it's good to say 'sup to your skin and see what's new: A flaky nose bridge? A rough and bumpy chin? An itchy, scaly patch above your right eye? The sooner you catch things like these, the sooner you can treat them and prevent them from spreading.

Charlotte's Skin Chart: What's Your Type?

Signs You Have NORMAL Skin

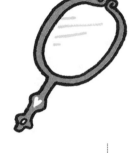

- You have little pores along the T-zone
- You rarely experience breakouts
- You experience a slight oily shine at the end of the day
- You rarely are sensitive to products

Here's the deal: You've basically hit the skin jackpot. Almost anything you put on your face, whether it has a heavy, medium, or light consistency or a formulation that's more oil-in-water or water-in-oil, is going to work fine for you. You've also probably skated through life with few blemishes, and your skin is relatively soft, bright, and firm.

Skin-care focus: Maintain and protect your healthy skin through cleansing, hydration, and sun protection.

Signs You Have DRY Skin

- You have very few visible pores and blackheads
- You have flaky or rough skin

- Your skin constantly feels tight or itchy
- You don't experience an oily shine

Your skin is flaky and rough and it needs to be nourished! Apply products with more of an oily, emollient base to protect your skin's barrier function. With your skin, you're more prone to visible signs of aging (fine lines and wrinkles). The upside of dry skin? You have small pores, you don't have to deal with an oil slick forehead, and you rarely have blemishes or acne.

Skin-care focus: Be vigilant about moisturizing and hydrating. Look for humectants that will bring back moisture to the skin and support a healthier barrier function.

Signs You Have OILY or ACNE-PRONE Skin

- You frequently experience breakouts and blackheads
- You have dilated or enlarged pores across the face
- You experience an oily shine and can feel oily residue when you touch your skin
- You are currently experiencing a breakout

Unlike your dry-skinned counterparts, your skin has lots of oil. This means your barrier function will be protected with natural oils, so you'll be looking youthful for longer. Unfortunately, excess oil also means the danger of acne breakouts! Gel creams (water-based formulas) work well with your skin type. Also, oil cleansers work wonders to gently remove sebum in the morning and at night.

Skin-care focus: Avoid clogged pores and control oil production by exfoliating with an ingredient such as salicylic acid. Use lightweight gel-type, water-based products to keep from adding oil to your skin and avoid emollients such as shea butter and lanolin. Finish off with oil-free makeup.

Cleansing is important here, especially if you have acne-prone skin. Use a gentle oil cleanser to remove your natural sebum. Don't use harsh exfoliators (with granules) over active breakouts. You'd benefit from anti-inflammatory and antibacterial ingredients such as tea tree oil. Make sure you protect with sunscreen, as acne eruptions are technically wounds and are subject to post-inflammatory pigmentation, meaning that they can darken permanently from sun exposure.

Signs You Have HORMONAL ACNE

- Your acne doesn't respond to topical treatments
- Your acne is primarily below the cheekbones and underneath the jaw
- Your acne is cystic, which means pimples are deeply embedded in the skin and painful
- Your acne flares up the week before or the week of your period

If you think this might be your case, talk to your dermatologist about having your hormone levels checked, or speak to an herbalist or nutritionist who can help you identify lifestyle tweaks to help find balance in your body and skin.

Signs You Have *COMBINATION* Skin

- You have visible pores along your T-zone (nose, forehead, and even some on your cheeks)
- You are oily around the T-zone, but rough and dry elsewhere
- Your skin is really indecisive—you've had to deal with flaky, dry patches and acne at the same time

Skin-care focus: Don't be afraid to use targeted treatments for different areas of your face. If you have an oily T-zone, use a BHA exfoliator and lightweight gel-type moisturizer there and a creamier, oil-based moisturizer in the dryer areas.

Signs You Have *SENSITIVE* Skin

- Your skin burns or itches when exposed to certain products or environments
- Your skin turns red or becomes bumpy easily

I would recommend making sure the products you use don't contain fragrances or dyes, both of which can be irritating. Avoid products that are highly alkaline and strong chemical exfoliators. Also, if you can, first do a patch test of a product on your arm before purchasing.

Skin-care focus: Whether your skin is oily or dry, your first priority is to find gentle skin-care products that don't contain added fragrances or abrasive scrubs to avoid breakouts, redness, and irritation.

Now . . . What Products Do You Buy for Your Skin Type?

Whether you're at your local store or browsing online, you'll be confronted by an intimidating number of different brands with beautiful, colorful bottles competing for your attention. What's the first thing to consider? You're going to need a clean canvas. This means that you need to go in with no preconceived notions about skin care. It's time to bust some myths about skin care that are the result of years of marketing mumbo jumbo.

The Price

It's simply not true that the most expensive product is the best skin-care product. The beauty market in Korea is proof that you can buy well-formulated goods at really affordable prices. Sometimes the expensive brands are expensive not because of the ingredients they're using or because of the research that goes into their products, but because they have a huge marketing and celebrity spokesperson budget they have to recoup.

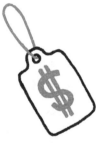

Your Sex

Boys, your only option is *not* a male skin-care line. I smile when a girl-friend tells me that her boyfriend uses her skin-care products. Dave and I frequently use the same products, and it's completely fine because, again, guys should also be purchasing based on skin type (not by a bottle saying that the product is for men!).

It's true that some men may have a bit more dry, irritated skin around the mouth and chin from shaving facial hair. There are even those who say men produce more oil than women, but in general, skin is skin and not everyone fits in a mold. Most of the time, the only difference is in the packaging and fragrance. Some dudes just want manlier-looking and -smelling products on their shelves, and that's fine—it's just good to know your options aren't that limited.

Your Age

Nope! Don't go there. Many people believe their age is the most important factor when deciding what products to try. The right products for you are not formulated by what age you are, but what conditions you see on your skin. Are all forty-year-olds dealing with the same skin issues? Nope. So you shouldn't buy a line based on what age group you belong to, case closed. Age ain't nothing but a number.

Dermatologist Recommended

It sounds legit and official, but this phrase can be used even if only one dermatologist gives a product a thumbs-up—and that dermatologist could have been paid for the endorsement. The assurance we get that a product has been backed by a doctor undoubtedly has some sway, but don't be tricked into thinking it means the product is magical or somehow right for you.

Hypoallergenic

This word is commonly found on products that claim to produce fewer allergic reactions. But there are currently no FDA regulations for hypo-allergenic formulas, so a company can use the term however it pleases! Sorry, sensitive skin types, you don't have it easy—it's better for you to learn what irritants cause you to break out and avoid them by looking at the ingredients list on the back of the bottle. Even dermatologists say the term has very little meaning.

Cosmeceutical

Another sneaky term, it means the product has drug or medicinal benefits, but the FDA has no regulations in place, so again anyone can slap that claim on a bottle. If it really, truly had medicinal benefits, then it would be a drug, not a cosmetic. If you come across anything that's labeled as a "hypoallergenic dermatologist-recommended cosmeceutical," you've basically hit the skin-care b.s. jackpot.

Natural, "Chemical-Free" Products

It sounds mighty appealing to go for all-natural skin care, but is it truly better? In a perfect world, every natural ingredient is better for you than synthetic, but we live in an imperfect world where plenty of natural things are extremely irritating to skin! Take poison ivy, for example, or even just grass! Many synthetic preservatives work better to stabilize the product and are effective in preserving it for longer periods of time. If you are gung-ho about using an all-natural formula that is preservative-free, be aware that its shelf life will be incredibly short, and you might have to chuck it before you've had a chance to use it up.

On that note, chemical-free products are highly sought after. I know the word "chemical" sounds scary, but did you know that you yourself are made up of millions and millions of chemicals? So it's not black and white. The best recommendation is always to understand what ingredients work and don't work for you.

> *When should you throw out products?*

Skin-care products don't last forever. Oxygen, water, and bacteria from your icky fingers digging around the jar all make sure of that. Look for the period-after-opening (PAO) symbol of a little open jar on the packaging and you'll see a number next to an "M" that signifies how many months a product is good for after it's been opened. While every product you use will differ (especially if it's in jar packaging vs. pump), my personal rule is that skin-care products should be thrown out within one year after they've been open. Attention, hoarders: Products that have not been opened will be stable for two to three years.

#SoKoSecret: Many Korean brands put the manufacturing date on their products instead of the expiration date. Sometimes people freak out when they see this date and think, This product is already expired! As Korean brands become more global, some have started to switch to the expiration date method. If you see the Korean characters "제조" after the date, that means the date signifies the manufacturing date, not the expiry.

> *Is it okay to mix and match brands?*

Absolutely. Never feel as if you have to use one line to get the best results (that's a popular marketing tactic, so don't fall for it!). There have been so many cases, in my experience, where a certain brand has an amazing facial oil but a terrible moisturizer. Mix and match to your skin's content.

> *Why Korean products?*

I would never say you have to use Korean beauty products in order to get healthier, more youthful-looking skin. As I've said before, many Western products are popular in Korea. What is most important is arming yourself with the right knowledge and investigating the proper product for you. It might be that it's made in Korea, or it might not.

But there's a reason so many beauty trends and products made in Korea are influencing the world in terms of product offerings and even key ingredients. The country is incredibly beauty focused and has a knowledgeable consumer base that has transformed the industry as a whole, keeping companies on their toes to meet the demand for impressive, high-quality products. Here are some of the reasons why Korea is a leader in skin care and beauty:

The ABCs of Skin-Care Shopping

- *Great formulas with affordable prices.* Koreans are serious about their skin care. They know what they want and how they want it, and they don't want to pay a fortune for it. That makes Korean cosmetic companies work harder to create only the best products at reasonable price points. That's why large global cosmetic companies look to the Korean consumer market to test their products. If it does well in Seoul, it'll do well elsewhere.

- *Innovative research and development.* As explained above, Korean cosmetic companies really value consumer opinions, so there's an intense focus on research and development to satisfy customers' stringent standards and needs. The result? An explosion of cutting-edge and effective products such as cushion compacts, sheet masks, and fermented skin-care products.

- *New and powerful ingredients.* As I said before, it's not about price, it's about well-formulated products that are gentle yet effective. Korean consumers consistently provide feedback that they have sensitive

#SoKoSecret: Fermented skin care is the latest in Korean skin-care innovation. Fermenting skin-care ingredients is beneficial because the process of converting fruits, plants, herbs, and yeast yields skin-loving amino acids and antioxidants that absorb more easily. Brands like Su:m37 and Goodal focus on using fermented ingredients in their formulas.

skin, so the companies focus on using well-tested and nourishing ingredients to moisturize and treat skin. It's not about immediate results, but consistent use that will bring skin to a healthier state.

- *Well-designed products that look awesome.* Korean cosmetic companies have really upped the ante on aesthetically pleasing packaging and design, and you'll find everything from *gwiyeowo* ("cute") to sophisticated elegance. If you're going to use a product every morning and night, it might as well look pleasing to the eye and it sure makes skin care and beauty as enjoyable as it is beneficial! Again, companies look to consumer feedback to see how they can improve the user experience. They're willing to be creative and take risks, so cue the panda hand cream.

Want to hear about my favorite brands? Head on over to chapter eleven for a complete guide to skin-care shopping in Seoul!

Ingredients to Be Excited About

Ingredient	What It Is	What It Does
Hyaluronic Acid	Humectant, moisturizer	Adds moisture
Glycerin	Humectant, moisturizer	Adds moisture
Honey	Anti-inflammatory, antioxidant	Heals wounds, fights signs of aging
Ceramides	Moisturizer	Restores moisture, improves skin texture
Urea	Humectant, moisturizer	Adds moisture
Glycolic Acid	Chemical exfoliant (AHA), humectant	Exfoliates, adds moisture, brightens skin
Lactic Acid	Chemical exfoliant (AHA), humectant	Exfoliates, adds moisture, brightens skin, reduces wrinkles
Kojic Acid	Melanin inhibitor	Decreases hyperpigmentation
Niacinamide	Antioxidant, melanin inhibitor	Fights free radicals; hydrates; improves elasticity; decreases hyperpigmentation, redness, and fine lines/wrinkles
Salicylic Acid	Chemical exfoliant (BHA), anti-inflammatory, antibacterial	Removes sebum, treats acne
Benzoyl Peroxide	Antibacterial	Treats acne

Mandelic Acid	Chemical exfoliant (AHA)	Decreases hyperpigmentation, exfoliates, adds moisture
Vitamin A	Antioxidant	Treats acne, reduces wrinkles, decreases hyperpigmentation
Vitamin C (other forms: calcium ascorbate, ascorbic acid, ascorbyl palmitate, Ester-C)	Antioxidant, melanin inhibitor	Stimulates collagen production, adds moisture, brightens skin
Vitamin E	Antioxidant	Adds moisture, decreases hyperpigmentation, fights free radicals
Caffeine	Antioxidant	Reduces redness, fights free radicals
Red Raspberry Extract	Antioxidant, antibacterial	Reduces redness
Zinc Oxide	Physical sunscreen	Protects from UVA and UVB rays
Titanium Dioxide	Physical sunscreen	Protects from UVA and UVB rays
Ginseng	Antioxidant	Stimulates collagen production
Snail Secretion Filtrate	Moisturizer	Hydrates, stimulates collagen production
Saccharomyces Ferment Filtrate	Antioxidant, anti-inflammatory	Hydrates, fights signs of aging, brightens skin
Green Tea	Antioxidant	Hydrates, fights signs of aging
Tea Tree Oil	Antibacterial, anti-inflammatory	Treats acne

• •

So it's time to start shopping. But before you begin, remember to be wary of falling into the trap of believing that a particular product will magically give you perfect skin. Keep in mind it takes time to see results. That means being knowledgeable about ingredients and using the products you need to consistently support your skin's natural defenses and improve whatever conditions you see. The goal here is not perfect skin—there is no such thing as perfect skin!—but to get your skin the healthiest it can be.

Even in Seoul, when I see someone whose dewy complexion looks flawless, I just remind myself that it probably just *looks* perfect. She might have blackheads on her nose, a flaky chin, and a shiny forehead, but she knows what to do and what to use to control it. Just like you. So let's go shopping.

SKIN STORIES: Paul Kang

SENIOR VICE PRESIDENT OF AMOREPACIFIC'S SKINCARE RESEARCH DIVISION

In the United States, skin care accounts for about 20 percent of the beauty market, but in Korea, it's more around 50 percent. Prevention is the biggest segment of skin care in Korea. Consumers are of two minds: They hope that products will work to treat and correct, but don't really expect them to work miracles and turn back time, so they focus a lot on preventing skin problems before they appear. Korean consumers really believe that they will see big results if they continually care for their skin for a long time.

Consumers don't care what information we put on the bottle about what a product does. Instead, they will look for reviews on the Internet, or listen to what their friends are saying about a product and then test it themselves. The makeup category is growing in Korea, and a lot of that is consumers wanting products that do more than one thing—like cushion compacts, which is makeup that also protects the skin. Korean women spend a lot of time and effort on skin care, but they want their makeup routine to be as quick and easy as possible.

The two most important determining factors in what products you should use are your genetic makeup—your skin type—and your climate. People in California will use different products from people in Singapore. A lot of Koreans have sensitive skin, so even when something is formulated and tested on Caucasian skin, it can still be irritating for a lot of Koreans. And even though our consumers want antiaging products, they still want them to be very safe. If they are not satisfied with a new product, then it is gone.

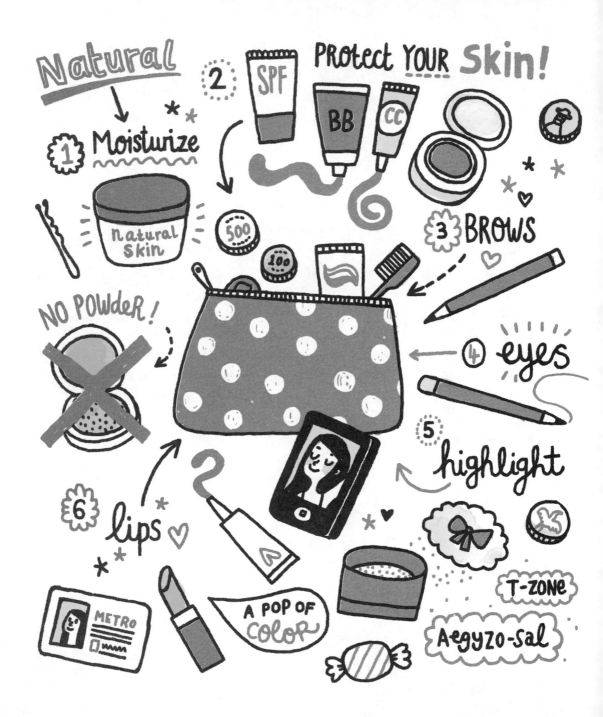

Putting Your Best Face Forward:

Fashion and No-Makeup Makeup

When I moved to Korea, one of the first things I noticed was that the women always looked so put together. Even if they were just going to the 7-Eleven to buy a pack of pads, their hair, clothes, and shoes would be completely on point. Or it could be snowing, and I'd peer out the bus window to see a woman in heels trudging—er, delicately stepping— through the snow to get to work. How was she going to last all day in a pair of wet pumps?

This was the opposite of my approach. I could clean up nice, but the rest of the time, who cares? I'd gladly walk in a Starbucks with tweaked- out bedhead and sweats that I'd slept in and stand in line behind a bunch of girls who looked pretty much the same. Even for Angelenos and New Yorkers, the concept of trying to look good at all times is foreign.

Growing up, I remember a blowout family fight before a trip to Hawaii. My mom insisted that my brother change out of his sweatpants and into jeans because we were "going to the airport." I sided with my brother because I had my own plans to wear sweats and wanted be as comfortable as possible on that long 6 A.M flight.

It seemed bizarre to me that my mom would want us to be presentable when we were just going to curl up and go to sleep, but after living in Korea, I came to understand that caring about appearance was part of her heritage. Korean culture cares a lot about doing and being your best. Whether it's career, academics, or personal achievements, people want to know that they gave it their all, and it's natural that this would trickle into how you look: They want to put their best face forward. Literally.

Korea is also a fast-fashion and fashion-forward culture. You could be forgiven for spending hours online looking at Seoul street-style blogs, or getting caught gawking on the street at some girl whose outfit you're trying to memorize so you can copy it later.

Trend spotting is relatively easy in Seoul, because when a trend hits, *everyone* is taking part. Compared with the population of the United States (which was 319 million as of 2014), Korea is tiny, with just 51 million people, but more than 10 million—roughly 20 percent of the country—reside in Seoul. That's more people in one place than in New York City (8.5 million), and the metropolitan population of Seoul is the second largest in the world after Tokyo. The concentration of people in Seoul makes for a remarkably urban and sophisticated culture on the whole, and one that's constantly hungry for the next big thing. When a trend is sparked by a celebrity's new lip color or haircut, it's very apparent that something's happening, because you'll see girls rocking it every which way you turn. When actress Ko Joon Hee came out with a short bob in a drama, so did many of my colleagues that season. I even wondered if I should take the plunge and get the cut myself.

Korean companies are also experts at fast-tracking trendy products to market, both in beauty and in fashion, so you can see something on a popular drama or on the runway and add a much cheaper version to your closet just a month or two later. I hate having the same things as other people, but when you see it that often, you start to experience a bit of fashion FOMO. I know, I know—that's not the deepest thing I've ever said, but I'm being honest here.

When I'm in New York, the threads I wear that get the most compliments are all things I got from Korean boutiques. Italian men have complimented my flats and women in SoHo have asked me where I got my jacket. Some were shocked when I mentioned it was from a small boutique in Seoul, but those more familiar with Korean fashion always responded with "Of course it is, I should have guessed!"

So Korea does have fashion down, with the cutest clothes sans expensive prices, but such fast fashion does have its downsides. The biggest is that many stores are one-size-fits-all, (meaning small), which isn't very inclusive and can make anyone who's not that one size feel pretty darn inadequate. Seoul is currently experiencing an influx of foreign stores such as Forever 21, H&M, and Zara, and these stores are having a good influence in the size department; some local lines are increasing their size range.

Putting Your Best Face Forward

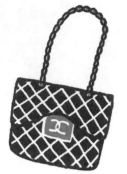

I was never a brand whore before coming to Korea, but a few years after I arrived, I must have blacked out while shopping. When I came to, I was the semi-proud owner of a (totally over my budget) Chanel flap bag. My colleagues, who knew that I once despised the luxury-brand game, teased me relentlessly. "You've become fully Korean," they said, and when I went home, my sister joked that Korea had changed me. But I quickly changed back, and the Chanel now sits in its dust bag, gathering dust. So as much as some parts of Korean culture rubbed off on me, there are others that just didn't stick—and my bank account is pretty thankful for that.

The Elephant in the Room: Plastic Surgery in Korea

I want to address the topic of plastic surgery in Korea, because you've likely heard about it already, and Korea has the highest per capita rate of cosmetic surgeries in the world. One of my pet peeves is the belief, popular outside of Asia, that surgery is done to look more Western and less Asian. I don't believe this is the whole story or the main factor. Instead, I think the popularity of plastic surgery comes from Korean culture's pressure to strive for and achieve perfection.

All cultures value attractiveness, but with a rising economy, money to spend, and a highly competitive atmosphere, Korean men and women find it necessary to invest in plastic surgery to remain in the game. Beauty, like wealth or social status, is a privilege that grants its owner many advantages.

I personally have no problem with plastic surgery. But as with any beauty procedure or treatment, plastic surgery becomes a problem when it's no longer done in moderation. For example, if someone is prioritizing cosmetic procedures over necessary health care, spending beyond their budget, or obsessing about completely changing the way they look, then any of these could be a sign that they're at risk for taking it too far.

I think it's a healthier and better option to invest in and partake in the Korean mindset of skin care. Skin care is noninvasive and less expensive, and clear, healthy skin makes people feel and look better. And they still get to look like themselves!

Gender Equality in Skin Care

Korean men are just as meticulous as women when it comes to their appearance. Many times I've been in a salon—from an expensive one in Cheongdam-dong for a cut and color to a local, more affordable chain for a blow out—and looked around to find myself outnumbered by men five to one. Heads deep in the shampoo bowls to my right *and* left, men.

If you've ever wondered how or why Korean men have the most awesome heads of hair, it's because they really do invest a lot of time and money in it. For example, man perms are pretty popular. But before you think *NSYNC-era Justin Timberlake curls, it's really more of a body wave, which adds a little volume to otherwise very straight hair. You probably wouldn't even notice it unless you were deliberately looking for it.

*Putting Your
Best Face
Forward*

Instead, you'd just spot some guy with a fabulous head of hair and think, *Swoon. What a hunk!*

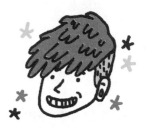

Korean men have a greater appetite for cosmetics and skin care than their American counterparts, and the general (non-dancing and -singing) male population in Seoul is well versed in skin care. Most Korean brands have lines of men's products, which are often very similar to the standard line, but tweaked with guy-friendly packaging and fragrances. All young men in Korea do mandatory military service (they serve from twenty-one to twenty-four months), and some brands even have products specifically targeted to military men—think skin-friendly camo war paint with a built-in SPF and special wipes to remove it. Skin-care stores that deliberately set up shop near military bases are usually bustling and probably would not be a bad place to hang out if you're a single lady looking for love.

Hellen Choo, the founder and CEO of Swagger (a Korean male cosmetics line) confirmed that a lot of Korean men are also not afraid to add a BB cream or tinted moisturizer to their routine to help even out their skin tone, especially before important events like job interviews or dates.

Meet Your New Beauty Icons: Korean Air Flight Attendants

I noticed it first on my Korean Air flight from Los Angeles to Seoul. I was *not* wearing sweatpants (my mom's pleading for her children to look nice at the airport finally sank in), and my flight started off business as usual. I bumped my way down the aisle, looking for my seat, while hoping there was still room for my carry-on in the overhead and keeping my fingers crossed that the person sitting next to me wouldn't be a creep who tried to make small talk for thirteen hours.

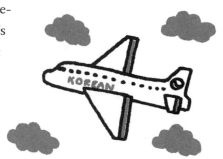

Score! I found a space in the overhead, and as I struggled to hoist my suitcase up, a soft, singsongy voice offered to help me. I gratefully accepted, and as I turned, I was immediately in awe of a beautiful woman with a peaceful smile and not a hair out of place. Not only was I impressed with how she handled my bag as if it weighed only five pounds, but her porcelain skin was absolutely radiant.

I sank into my seat with my mouth slightly open and blatantly stared—I guess the creep on this flight was me. When I went to the bathroom, there was a bottle of something called "essence" next to the sink, and when I returned to my seat, the woman next to me was already in full-on sheet mask glory. Hmm, I thought. I'm no dummy—*something* was going on here.

The attendant who had helped me wasn't the only one who was

glowing—the entire cabin crew looked downright ethereal. Spending hours in drying atmospheres and breathing recycled air was a huge part of their jobs, so how did they keep it up? On domestic American flights, the crew always looked a little more haggard, and with that much travel, who could blame them? But everyone who worked for Korean Air had a crisp uniform; hair in a tight, low bun with a blue pin (a Korean Air trademark); black shoes with a low, chunky heel; and smooth, clear skin. And other than a slight pink tint to the lips, it looked as if they were wearing hardly any makeup—definitely no caked-on foundation. This "no-makeup makeup" look seemed effortless and natural, yet polished and miles away from my own no-makeup days. I wanted to know all their secrets: What skin-care products did they use? What was in their makeup bags? (If I'd known where they were stowed, I would have snuck a peek during meal service.) But could it just be products? Maybe there was something in the water . . .

#SoKoSecret If you're traveling, a good way to combat low humidity in airplanes is regularly spritzing with a facial mist that contains humectants, which will help keep you hydrated. Keep in mind that facial sprays that are just water will actually dehydrate your skin even more.

Pack Your Makeup Bags

I'd soon come to find that although Korean Air flight attendants go through strict makeup classes for appearance and etiquette, this "no-makeup

makeup" look was everywhere in Seoul. A few months later, I finally learned how to re-create it for myself. There are some subtle techniques involved, but they're easy to master. Here's the basic equipment you need to pull it off—no life vest or seat belts required.

The BB Cream

An all-in-one moisturizer with a tinted color for coverage, BB cream, was created in Germany. It was originally a formula to help moisturize and cover up postsurgical scars, but women soon started to discover and appreciate its cosmetic uses—especially Korean women, who were frustrated with the makeup options already on the market.

Traditional foundation covered stuff up, but its positive qualities ended there. It often appeared flaky and caked on and felt like wearing a coat of paint. To add insult to injury, it also dried skin out and wasn't good for your skin, which definitely did not jibe with Koreans' skin-first philosophy. Korean cosmetic companies took the original concept of BB cream and evolved it into something that would cover up imperfections, but also prep and moisturize while providing antiaging and brightening properties and sun protection.

Now almost every cosmetics company (not just Korean) has added a BB cream to its line, but not all are created equal. Some are just modified foundations, without the beneficial ingredients or effects, so read the label carefully. Unfortunately, there's not much shade variation in Korean skin tone, so many companies don't offer a huge range of shades. However, this is changing, and more companies with an eye on the global market are stepping it up.

My picks:

Missha M Perfect Cover BB Cream is what put the brand Missha on the map. It blends naturally, evens out skin tone, and creates a flawless finish, all with SPF 42/PA+++.

Skin79 Super+ Beblesh Balm Triple Functions has Korean beauty cult status. For light skin tones, this BB offers brightening, antiaging properties with SPF 25/PA++.

Klairs Illuminating Supple Blemish Cream is a light and nongreasy formula that delivers skin-hydrating benefits with hyaluronic acid, aloe, and SPF 40/PA++.

The CC cream (or color correcting cream), offers the same benefits as the BB such as antiaging properties, hydration, SPF, and coverage, but goes on a little more sheer, is less heavy in consistency, and has a more natural look. CC creams vary from brand to brand, so this might not be the case for all CC creams on the market, but you can sample a few to find one that has the results you're looking for.

Now some companies are even offering DD creams (which typically stands for "daily defense") and such, but don't take them seriously unless you can actually see what makes the formula different. Innovation takes more than just marching down the alphabet, so a lot of these smell like a gimmick. A future ZZ cream would seem suspicious to me.

My picks:

Banila Co It Radiant CC Cream blends in seamlessly to hydrate, prime, conceal, and protect (SPF 30 PA++ broad spectrum) your skin. Leaves you with a radiant, glowing complexion that will last all day.

Banila Co. It Radiant CC Melting Foundation is a hydrating CC and foundation duo with SPF 32/PA++ that blends in creamy but finishes lightweight and matte.

The Cushion Compact

The cushion compact is an upgrade to the form and application of a BB cream. The formula has all the properties (coverage, antiaging, brightening, hydrating, moisturizing, and SPF protection), but the application and tool used in the compact allows for a very sheer, natural application. Developed in 2007 by researchers at AmorePacific, the cushion compact solved several makeup problems in one fell swoop: It was easy to carry, went on lighter than cake makeup, and wasn't drying like a powder. Now, it's estimated that an IOPE Air Cushion XP (the original) is sold every six seconds in Korea, and it's easy to see why: They're just freaking awesome.

The cushion that holds the makeup is specially designed not to dry out (even if you accidentally leave it open sometimes, like I do) and the applicator sponge is designed to not absorb the makeup, which means more goes on the skin. It's incredibly easy and fast to apply—you tap the applicator on the cushion, then tap it on your skin—and to retouch throughout the day because it isn't a heavy cream. The makeup itself is lightweight and usually formulated with an SPF of 30 or above. Plus, it just gives you a glow—and that's what this is all about, right?

My picks:

IOPE Air Cushion XP is the first and original cushion compact (in the world!). The cooling, refreshing formula is SPF 50+/PA+++ and can be applied at the start of your makeup routine and throughout the day for a dewy, hydrated glow.

AmorePacific Color Control Cushion Compact also delivers a flawless, luminous complexion. Its superstar antioxidant ingredient, green tea, brightens and hydrates, and the product has SPF 50+ broad spectrum protection.

Banila Co. VV Bouncing Cushion provides full coverage of blemishes, fine lines, and uneven skin tone without cakiness and finishes off with silky matte coverage with SPF 50+/PA+++. The formula is dispensed using the brand's Mega Pump Up System—just push down on the circular rim for the foundation to appear.

Want to stick to something with more coverage? Try these foundations.

Son & Park Skin Fit Foundation is such an innovative approach to foundation because it's in stick form and has essence in the center of its formula! Plus, it offers sun protection of SPF 45/PA++.

Son & Park Air Chou Foundation applies on creamy and finishes off with a natural, matte finish. The light coverage leaves skin looking bright and soft all day long. Recommended for combination to oily skin types.

The Eyeliner

Koreans are obsessed with having very bright eyes, and some girls even wear "big-eye" contact lenses, which enlarge the irises to almost anime proportions. But the easier, more comfortable, everyday staple is eyeliner. They use gel pots, pen liners, liquid liners, and pencils, but it's ever present and almost always black or brown. And rather than a sweeping cat eye or a heavily lined lower lid, it's usually a subtle look that follows the natural shape of the eye.

My picks:

Clio Waterproof Pen Liner has achieved holy grail eyeliner status. The brush-tip pen applicator allows for a precise line that lasts all day and night, and it's easy to remove with an oil cleanser or makeup remover.

Clio Gelpresso Pencil Gel Liner is a versatile, long-wearing shimmery and creamy eyeliner that glides on effortlessly.

Clio Gel Liner and Brow Pot is a creamy gel liner and brow powder duo that ensures all-day wear. It comes conveniently packaged with a two-sided brush for brow and eyeliner application.

The Eyebrow Pencil

I've always had little stubby, fuzzy caterpillar eyebrows because I take after my dad. He looks as if he has two monarch butterflies about to hatch on his forehead (sorry, Dad, love you!). I've had to shape and elongate them for as long as I can remember, and I normally don't leave the house without drawing them in.

In high school, they looked like they were Sharpied in, because I was always trying to emulate the thin arches I'd see on celebrities. But in Korea, women avoid overplucking and dramatic shapes and focus instead on enhancing the natural shape they have. Also, thick, full eyebrows can make you look more youthful, while drawn-on arches can add years to your face.

I've learned that the trick to eyebrows is making sure I'm not just going with a shape that's trendy, but one that is actually pleasing with my face and eyes. Makeup trends come and go, but they're not as cyclical as fashion, and they require more personalization to get them right.

My picks:

Lioele Artist Eyebrow Pencil is an all-in-one eyebrow pencil with a retractable pencil and brow brush that helps fill in your brows for a natural, full look.

Innisfree Eco Design Eyebrow Pencil is the ultimate eyebrow pencil that you never have to sharpen. Twist to reveal the angled tip and use it to reshape and define your brows naturally.

The Faceshop Lovely ME:EX Design My Eyebrow is another eyebrow pencil that twists up and has a sturdy spoolie on the other end to brush away harsh lines for a natural, full brow.

The Lip Tint

The actresses on Korean dramas have a way of sparking a beauty trend and making it spread like wildfire. In some cases, these trends go global and aren't even about Korean-branded items. *My Love from Another Star* was a hugely popular Korean drama about a real star (as in fell from the heavens and now lives on Earth) who falls in love with a celebrity star, played by actress Jeon Ji Hyun. She wore a certain lip color from Iope, and it sold out globally after the episode aired. Within days, the only ones available were on eBay with jacked-up prices (no thanks!).

Korean girls also tend to eschew a heavy lip in favor of tints and stains, and a vivid lip (whether it is perfectly manicured or smudged as if you sucked on a pink lollipop) makes your clean, clear skin look even brighter.

#ᏚᎧᏦᎧᏚᏋᏟᏒᏋᏖ Lip stains applied in the center (as in a gradient lip) are so popular because it draws the eye to the fullest part of the lip and makes the wearer look younger.

My picks:
Son & Park Air Tint Lip Cube a vibrant and creamy tint that has a matte finish.

3CE Water Tint boosts your natural lip color with a pigment-rich tint and creates a moisturizing layer to lock in the moisture.

Son & Park Lip Crayon is a playful fusion between lipstick and lip tint.

Tony Moly Petite Bunny Gloss Bar is a gloss with a slight tint, a fruity flavor, and tons of moisture. Bonus: bunny ear packaging.

The Highlighter
No, not a bright yellow marker, but a pearly, dusty shadow or a shimmery, pearlized cream that catches the light. A highlighter adds dimension to the face and helps create that dewy glow. Yes, it's true: You want a naturally dewy glow, but you can also enhance it with a bit of highlighting.

Although women in Korea do use contouring to make the jaw, and face as a whole, look smaller, it isn't overdone. Shading can look heavy and like a throwback to our mothers' generation, and that, my friends, is not the goal. Instead, a little highlighter helps draw attention to the parts of your face that are naturally the slimmest and the areas that you want to, um, highlight.

So to start, first dab the highlighter on the areas the sunshine naturally hits, like the tops of the cheekbones, bridge of the nose, chin, and forehead, then a bit under the eyes. I know, you're probably like, "Under the eyes? Um, no way am I highlighting my bags." But hear me out: The Koreans actually have a term—*aegyo-sal*—for the cute little "pudge" that shows up under your eyes when you're smiling. A dab of highlighter under the eyes not only brightens them, but also can actually help you look cheerful and bright even when you're totally pissed off.

So the next time your boss asks you to come in on a Saturday, just excuse yourself, take your highlighter to the bathroom, then come back and say, "No problem!" Your eyes will be smiling even if you aren't.

My picks:

Son & Park Highlighter Cube preps your face for a glowing, fresh look. It's iridescent, with hints of coral that will make your skin naturally luminous.

Etude House Dear Girls Big Eyes Maker is a light champagne-pink highlighter used to line underneath and the inner corners of the eyes for a bright, youthful look.

3CE Highlight Beam is a creamy illuminator that's great for highlighting your cheeks, brow bones, nose, and even neck and shoulders.

The Toothbrush (And No, It's Not for Brushing Brows)

In Korea, oral hygiene is not just a morning and night deal. In offices, such as a doctor's clinic or even mine at Samsung, there will be rows of toothbrushes lined up in the bathroom, with the entire staff stopping in to brush after lunch. It's normal to catch people brushing their teeth in a public restroom at school or in a shopping mall. And if someone doesn't have a little toothbrush and toothpaste set in her makeup bag, you probably won't have to look in too many other places to find it. It might even be stuck in the pencil holder on her desk. After all, you want your teeth to be in good shape so that they can pair with your perfect pink lips for a beautiful, beguiling smile.

The Techniques

Let me be clear: The "no-makeup makeup" look doesn't necessarily mean you apply less makeup (are you beauty addicts breathing a sigh of relief?). It just means that you use different products and different techniques, and that your final look doesn't come with a big, blinking arrow that says MAKEUP. Subtle is the name of the game.

Also, not every product and technique is going to work for everyone. You might not think a bright lip looks good on you, or your eyebrows might not require any touching up—awesome! Because your face is so uniquely you, you're going to be the expert on your own look, and it might take some trial and error to hit on what you like best. But that trial and error is going to be super fun, so here are a few tricks of the trade for figuring out what's the right look for you.

1. It all starts with the skin.

Your skin, and not a BB cream, is the true foundation of this look. You know that comprehensive, fully customizable skin-care routine that I went on and on about earlier? This is where it comes into play. You start there, because you want your skin to be prepped and moisturized properly before you even think about adding anything on top. Makeup keeps trending more and more natural, even in high fashion, which means that the importance of good skin isn't going to go away anytime soon.

2. Then comes the good-for-you foundation.

After you've added your moisturizer, you're going to want to protect your skin with sunscreen. Then dab on your BB cream, CC cream, or cushion compact (which will probably have SPF as well).

When I'm using a cushion compact, I start at the center of my face (my nose) and work out, because you want the outside to be the most natural to avoid a visible line where the makeup stops. We've all seen women whose faces are a different color from their necks, and this shall not be you!

With creams, feel free to use your fingertips, a makeup brush, or a beautyblender-type sponge, but the application is the same. Start at the center, work out, and blend well at the edges.

3. Draw your eyebrows in, not on.

For brunettes, a general rule of thumb is to choose a pencil that's one shade lighter than your natural hair color. If you're a blonde or have light hair, do the opposite and choose a color that's one shade darker.

Fill in any sparse or undergrown areas from where your brows begin, in line with the edges of your nose (on the inside), to where they tail off. To find this ideal end point, imagine there's a diagonal line going from the bottom of your nose to the outside corner of your eye and then extending on to your hairline. Stop there.

4. All about the eyes.

Save the smoke for the Korean BBQ joints, because it has no place in this look. A smoky eye is the opposite of understated beauty, and the goal here is to keep everything as natural as possible and just enhance the shape of your eyes. If you want your eyes to look rounder, you can line the entire top lid, but you can start in the middle or more toward the outer edge if you want to elongate the shape. Draw on a thin line, and don't blend it.

Of course, long, lush eyelashes are a welcome addition to the eyes. Say hello to eyelash extensions. It's common to get them done in Seoul to keep the eyes looking lush while avoiding the eyelash curler and mascara. I've had them done several times, and they're especially great before photo shoots or events. I've even heard of women getting them when they're about to have a baby, so they don't look quite so bleary in delivery room photos!

5. Now we're on to the cheeks.

Instead of smiling hard and applying blush on the apples of your cheeks (as we were always told to do) to create a flushed look, take your shimmery highlighter and smooth it along the cheekbones, nose, and forehead. Basically, this is your T-zone and also the areas that the sun naturally hits. It's possible to get a little too highlighter happy and come out looking like a pearl, so use in moderation. Subtle is better, and dab a bit in the corners of and under your eyes for the aforementioned *aegyo-sal*.

6. The lips are the focal point of this look.

When they're bright and vivid, it's a good contrast and really shows off your beautiful skin. A pop of color is also good for all seasons, whether it's winter or summer. You can carefully paint on the tint within your natural lip line, or just dab it in the center of the lips, which will make you look like you just finished a strawberry Blow Pop. I love how easy this is to achieve. Your finger is literally the best tool for it, and it's a technique that's hard to mess up. Most teenagers don't even bother with blending—they just dab a dot in the center of their lips and call it a day. This look screams "I'm too cool and busy to even bother with a mirror" and is a sign of youth in makeup revolt.

7. This step is not a step.

It's all about skipping . . . the powder. In Korean beauty culture, powder has largely become a thing of the past. Unless they're extremely oily and need a powder to absorb some of the sebum, most Korean women don't bother with it. A heavy, matte look is the antithesis of the fresh and dewy look we're going for—which is not to be confused with shiny, of course.

8. Get dressed to impress.

Now that you're looking like you just "woke up like this," dress to impress for that *sogaeting*. Before online dating apps were popular, people filled their weekends with setups by mutual friends, and if they clean up nice to just run errands, you bet they pull out all the stops for their future significant others.

SKIN STORIES: Son Dae Sik

CEO OF SON & PARK AND OFFICIAL MAKEUP ARTIST FOR ACTRESS AND MODEL JEON JI HYUN

I believe that skin care is the most important part of your makeup routine. Without the proper prep, the condition of your skin has the potential to ruin your makeup for the day. I make sure to cleanse, then tone and exfoliate with the *Son & Park* Beauty Water to make sure my pores are cleansed properly. Then I apply serum. Last, I massage a light moisturizing cream into my skin for about three to five minutes. Massaging helps reduce swelling and helps the moisturizing ingredients penetrate.

The no-makeup makeup look is the look of choice in Korea right now, and this means using light and natural makeup to subtly enhance facial features. In theory it's an easy technique, yet the hardest to actually get right.

Although it depends on her outfit and hair, Jeon Ji Hyun prefers lighter makeup. I have to say, she does fit the natural, no-makeup makeup look best, so I keep myself from using too many color cosmetics and use just subtle contouring techniques to enhance her features. For the drama *Love from Another Star,* I focused on creating a clean, dewy look with a pop of color on the lips. She trusts me completely because she knows I will always make sure that her look is simply perfect.

*Putting Your
Best Face
Forward*

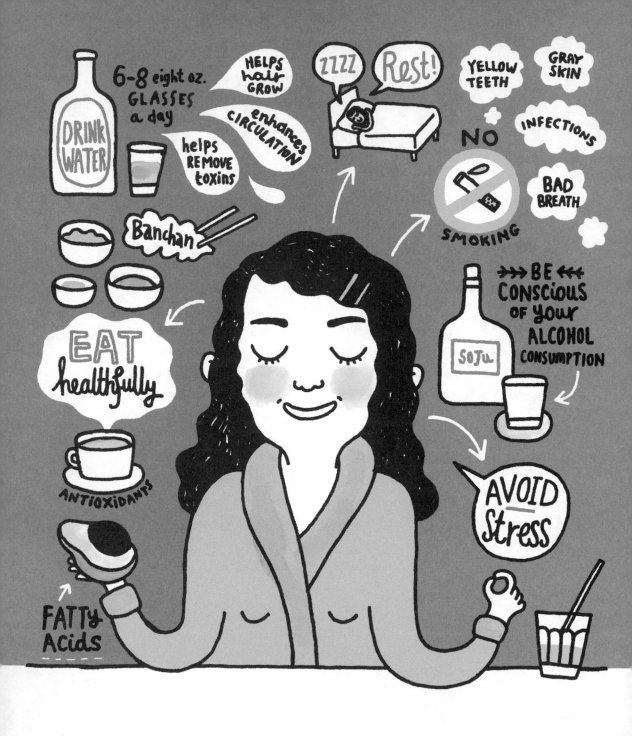

Korean Beauty from the Inside Out:

How Your Lifestyle Affects Your Skin

*I*n so many ways, when I moved to Seoul, I didn't know what to expect at all. One thing I wasn't worried about, though: stuffing my face. That was definitely going to happen, and I thoroughly looked forward to it.

Growing up in L.A., whether you wanted Korean BBQ, bibimbap, or copious amounts of kimchi, the local Korean restaurants did not disappoint. I'd always enjoyed Korean cuisine growing up, and seeking out the authentic versions of my favorite dishes was high on my Seoul bucket list.

But as much as I had a good handle on the grub and the chopsticks, there were still new culinary subtleties that I started to pick up on. For example, *banchan* was not just an amuse-bouche, much less decor for the

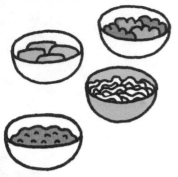

table, my aunt and uncle explained. Rather, it could make or break the main dish. The *banchan* served was so important to the harmony of the dish as a whole, they said, that if a restaurant specializing in oxtail soup didn't have good kimchi and *kkakdugi* (spicy radish) to pair with it, then that restaurant was surely not long for this world.

Since all *banchan* was not created equal, my palate soon developed so that I knew what was bomb *banchan* or just mediocre. Also, unlike spinach dip or an onion blossom, you could gorge on *banchan* and not feel a shred of guilt. You were just consuming lots of fresh and fermented veggies, an essential part of Korea's health-focused culture.

#SoKoSecret Many Korean people believe that fermented foods, such as kimchi, are rich in beneficial bacteria, powerful antioxidants, and enzymes that help with digestion and boost the immune system.

But the healthy effects of my new Korean lifestyle didn't stop at side dishes. When I worked at Samsung, my colleagues would ask me to join them on a walk along a landscaped trail that meandered not far from our office building. Originally, I interpreted these requests to be romantic gestures, but then I noticed that almost everyone in the company was out in pairs or small groups, walking off their lunch.

From yoga to hikes (which were taken seriously in head-to-toe professional hiking gear, not like L.A. hikes where you stroll up a hill in flip-flops) to eating right, Koreans seemed to take their overall well-being as seriously as they took their skin care.

Obviously, while not everything about Korean culture was the healthiest (like late-night soju-drinking sessions or the heavy pork belly consumption), it was still clear to me that many people—whatever their age or gender—made a concerted effort to be knowledgeable about what was good for them and took steps to invest in and care for their bodies. This wasn't a fad diet culture, as people seemed to understand and be okay with the fact that it might be twenty or thirty years before they reaped the benefits of what they were doing now. Instant gratification be damned—it will be worth it.

R-E-S-P-E-C-T Your Body

The basic truth: You can't respect your skin but trash your body and still expect to look radiant. I've said before that skin care is more than skin deep, and I'll say it again here. These are just a few tips for overall health that can have a major impact on your skin as well.

Drink a Lot of Water

Your body is about 60 percent water, so it makes sense that health authorities recommend drinking six to eight eight-ounce glasses a day (depending on if you exercise a lot). It keeps your immune system in tip-top shape, and it's hard to find a healthy complexion on an unhealthy body.

Water is also connected to our blood circulation, which helps keep skin looking bright and fresh. But don't overestimate the benefits of drinking water. I've heard this a million times: "I drink *so* much water. I don't know why my skin is still so dehydrated all the time!" Here's the deal: Water trickles down to your skin last. In other words, the water you drink is going to go to your kidneys, lungs, heart, and everything else first. You're not going to suddenly achieve plump, hydrated skin by drinking a lot of water, because our bodies are just not that simple. You get the best results when you drink enough water *and* hydrate your skin topically with humectants that bind moisture to the skin.

Eat Well

Your skin will mirror what you eat. Eating a balanced diet is the optimal way to keep your body healthy, and it will also be reflected on the outside. So eat less of those things that end in -os (Cheetos, Doritos, Haribos) and more yogurts, greens, fish, fruits, whole grains, and lean protein.

But as with drinking water, what you eat won't immediately improve your skin. Should you be eating an avocado or drinking green tea for the sake of your skin? Sure, the fatty acids and antioxidants are great sources of nutrition for your body as a whole. Like water, all the nutrients you get from food will be distributed to your vital organs first and then your skin. But in my book (and remember, this is my book!) this is just all the more reason to eat well, so that your mind and entire body (including your skin) are feeling nourished and in their optimal states.

Get Tons of Z's

Go ahead, knock yourself out: Sleeping is one of the best things you can do for your skin. From running Soko Glam to writing this book to watching

Running Man marathons (I can't help it! Have you seen this show?), I'm no stranger to sleep deprivation. When I don't get enough sleep, my body wastes no time in letting me know I've been very bad to it. I'm not as alert during the day and I get a lot of comments like, "Dude, you look *tired*." But aside from just being groggy and not that much fun when you're sleep deprived, the skin consequences range from puffy eyes to dark circles and even increased acne.

Why is getting seven to eight hours of deep sleep essential to your skin's health? While you rest, your body repairs itself. During sleep, blood flows toward the skin (rather than your body's core, as it does when you're awake), and it brings oxygen to the skin. Also, sleep is when amino acid molecules build more collagen and fluid and toxins are drained.

Now you're probably thinking about puffy eyes, which most of us have had to battle after pulling an all-nighter in college or a late-night job/school/boyfriend-related crying session. So what causes eyes to be puffy and, more important, how do we get rid of them?

While some of it can be hereditary (thank your parents), a lot of us do notice puffiness under the eyes after a night of tossing and turning. When we don't get enough sleep, or enough good sleep, excess fluid near the skin isn't transported to the bladder to be excreted; it sticks around in your face. There's less fat in the area right under your eyes, so water retention is more apparent, and dark circles are specifically the result of lack of blood flow to the skin.

Sleep deprivation also weakens the skin barrier function (the immune system that blocks out bad bacteria and other foreign substances), which can lead to skin disorders like eczema and accelerate signs of aging.

Reduce Stress

Aw, stress. A lot of us have been here: You have a weird ailment, your doctor takes your temperature, pokes and prods you, and then says definitively, "It's stress. You need to reduce your stress." And then you're just sitting there thinking, that can't be right.

But your doctor is right; stress is something that we all have to learn to manage. It can make a significant impact on your overall health, and in your skin it shows in things like breakouts and premature aging.

How stress affects your body breaks down like this: Stress (including trauma, pain, illness, or just an everyday situation) causes your body to release hormones such as adrenaline and cortisol, which are supposed to increase your energy and help you deal with whatever stressful situation is at hand. However, high levels of these hormones for a prolonged period of time weakens the epidermal barrier, which aggravates existing conditions or delays wound healing. When cortisol levels rise, sebaceous glands produce more oil. So this is why, when you're already stressed about trying to look your best—right before a date with a cute boy, or when you find out it will rain on your outdoor wedding—a big fat honker of a pimple decides to land on your nose.

Want proof? Look no further than our presidential figures. I'm teased a lot by my friends (and my husband) about my crush on President Obama. But after seven years in office, President Obama looks like he's aged twenty years—you can see gray hair, deep wrinkles, and skin that just looks less plump and more sallow. While I still think he's the cutest out of all our presidents, it's proof enough that stress can do a number on your skin. Obama might not get a chance to chill out anytime soon, but you should definitely do what you can.

The Surprising Upside of a Cultural Taboo

Being in a completely different country halfway across the world, you're bound to run into different mindsets and ways of living—you know, culture shock. Like using a bidet to wash your bum. At first it's gross if you're a newbie, but a few warm and satisfying squirts later, you're actually disgusted that you've lived your whole life without one.

In many ways, Korea is more conservative than the United States. Get addicted to a romantic Korean drama and you're going to be waiting a *loooonnnggg* time before the leads even kiss. After a few episodes, you start getting excited when it seems like they might hold hands! Premarital sex and living with your boyfriend are also still major social taboos, even though it's obviously done. With my Korean parents still in California, I figured it was safe for Dave and me to move in together in Seoul, then my dad called to announce he was coming to visit! Yay—but crap.

I went into panic mode. I leased a furnished apartment for a month, and Dave and I moved an entire carload of my stuff from the apartment that we shared to my new, pretend solo studio. Right before my dad was scheduled to arrive, he called me from LAX to let me know that he was checked in and that his flight was on time. "Oh, and Charlotte," he said before we hung up, "your mom wants to make sure you didn't rent a fake apartment so that we wouldn't know you're living with your boyfriend."

"No, of course not," I said, laughing. "Why would I do that?" With the month lease already signed, I had no choice but to just brazen it out and pretend that my parents didn't know exactly what I was up to. And let me tell you, a carload of stuff doesn't look like that much when it's all spread out in an apartment. When my aunt came to visit my dad and me at the apartment, she took one look around and said, "Where's all your stuff?" while my dad and I sat there, smiling and avoiding a bit of cross-continental confrontation.

While my parents were capable of surprising me, I was equally surprised by Korea as a whole. After I accepted the job at Samsung and gave my two weeks' notice, my American boss warned me to be careful and to be prepared for my opinions to not matter just because I was female. I brushed away his comments until I received my employment contract from Samsung. The fine print said that if I ever had a kid, I would have to be back in the office in three days after giving birth!

Holy shit! I thought. *They try to push you out as soon as you're a mom!* Maybe my boss was right, and I was transporting myself back to the 1950s, where I'd just serve coffee all day, no matter what my title. But I was twenty-two and felt light-years away from being affected by any pregnancy clause, so I signed.

Turns out the contract had a typo—there was a full three-month maternity leave with an option to extend if needed. Also, my opinions mattered a lot, and I was well rewarded for them. By my second year at Samsung, I was traveling on overseas business trips with Vice President Hong Sung Il and the CEO Park Ki Seok for exclusive meetings that I pitched and proposed. By twenty-four I received a special bonus from the company; by twenty-five I was making hiring decisions and managing million-dollar events; and by twenty-six I was leading the international public relations team. Shortly after I left Seoul in 2013, Korea elected its first female president.

My former boss was wrong in many ways, but there were a few lingering cultural taboos that women in Korea still had to face. One of them was smoking. Whereas no one would bat an eye if a guy were to pull out a pack, it was considered decidedly improper for a female to do so. I'd walk past cafés or drinking establishments and see huddles of Korean men drinking coffee and smoking, a large smoke cloud above them—and not a woman in sight. After a few years in Korea, even I became conditioned to do a double take if I saw a woman light up in public. Women still smoked, of course, but discreetly. In the bathroom of clubs, you'd fight your way to the mirror through groups of women chain-smoking safely out of public view.

I personally dig a sexy cigarette scene (thank you, Wong Kar Wai movies) and can see why smoking has such appeal. I've smoked a handful of times in my life—including a few to deliberately push the envelope with my colleagues while I was in Korea—but I never picked up the habit. And thank God.

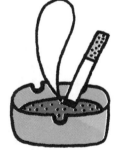

Now after diving deep into skin care, I'm even more grateful that my rebellious dalliances never led to a full-on habit, as it's occurred to me that this sexist smoking taboo has unintentionally helped Korean women avoid the pitfalls of smoking, which is one of the worst things you can do for your skin.

Here, let me create a visual for you. When you take that puff, smoke enters your body and your bloodstream and affects almost every organ in your body in the process. Smoke passes through your breathing tubes, or bronchi, which causes inflammation and coughing. You subject yourself to the potential for bronchial infections, lung cancer, and emphysema in your respiratory system, and gum disease and tooth decay in your mouth. Tobacco stains your teeth—mmm, yellow—and taints your breath. Nicotine raises your blood pressure and makes your blood clot, leading to cholesterol deposits on artery walls. Increased stomach acid secretions cause heartburn and ulcers, and carcinogens from the cigarette are excreted in your urine, which can cause bladder cancer and liver damage.

So there's that—now, on to your skin. Smoking reduces the amount of oxygen in your blood, and since blood flows to your skin last, the reduced oxygen starves skin cells and causes them to die off. Cellular turnover is slow, as cells are now dying as opposed to regenerating, and this leads to premature aging. Free radicals from cigarette smoke also cause cell damage and the breakdown of proteins. With less blood flow to your skin, your skin is less nourished, so skin tones can appear sallow and dull. It can also impact texture and smoothness. Furthermore, wounds are slower to heal, and you're at greater risk for skin cancer.

Drowning Your Sorrows Is Bad for Your Skin

Taboos usually come with a tinge of hypocrisy, and Korea is no different. As much as smoking is taboo for women, chugging the national spirit (soju) from the "green bottle" isn't. The green bottle is a big part of Korean culture. Sold readily at any convenience store for less than two bucks, soju has put Korea on the map for being the nation that drinks the most hard liquor: an average of 13.7 shots a week—twice the amount of Russia!

The biggest celebs in Korea—usually actresses—are frequently soju spokesmodels, with their faces even on the bottle, and the green bottle is a popular trope in movies and dramas. When rejected by a love, or facing similar hardships, an actor recounts his or her woes while dramatically downing shots either alone or with friends in a *pocha*, a tented outdoor bar established as a spot where people come to drink themselves into a drunken stupor. When they stumble home or into work the next morning, everyone politely turns the other cheek.

Alcohol is my vice of choice, and I made the most of my time in Seoul. I love soju and wine, and soju mixed with watermelon juice in particular is my weakness. But as fun as drinking (in moderation) can be, alcohol does a number on your body and causes blood vessels to expand and widen, allowing more blood to flow through your skin. While this might sound great, it's what creates that flush you get from drinking, and dilated blood vessels can lead to broken capillaries and a permanently ruddy complexion. High alcohol consumption also dehydrates your skin, increasing the appearance of fine lines. If you've ever looked in the mirror with a hangover and thought, *Oh man, one night of drinking aged me five years!*—bingo.

So while cutting out alcohol may be too much to ask, here are a few ways to decrease the impact of your consumption. One preventative measure is to make sure you moisturize your skin prior to drinking. Another is to opt for beer or wine (as a better alternative to spirits), and remember to take sips of water in between to keep you hydrated. After a night of drinking, it will be beneficial if you treat your face to a chilled sheet mask or a sleeping mask with vitamins and humectants for antioxidants and a hydration boost.

Boricha: Drink Up!

Go into any Korean household and you'll see *boricha* in the fridge next to a stack of *banchan* in clear glass containers. *Boricha* is a nutty-flavored, antioxidant-packed roasted barley tea that's chilled in the summer months and served warm in the winter. I'm convinced that diet contributes to a better body and better skin. Granted, there might not be a scientific study

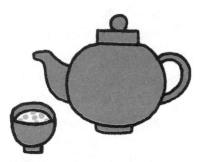

out there that explicitly connects the dots, but nonstop veggies + caffeine-free antioxidant tea = better health? Makes sense to me.

To make *boricha,* you can purchase loose barley grains and boil them in a pot for a few minutes before letting the mixture cool and transferring it to a pitcher. You can also buy barley tea bags that you pop into a pitcher and let soak for twenty minutes before discarding the bag.

Tea, though some contain caffeine, is also good for your skin, specifically green tea. It's packed with antioxidants and also has anticarcinogenic effects, whether you drink it or apply it topically to your skin. Green tea can help prevent collagen breakdown and keep UV rays from wreaking havoc on your skin, which has made it a hugely popular skin-care ingredient.

So when it comes to tea, drink it up and slather it on, and leave the soju on the shelf.

ORDER THIS: My Ten Favorite Korean Dishes

1. *Kimchi.* A spicy cabbage prepared with pepper, garlic, ginger, and scallions. It is a fermented *banchan* that's present at almost every meal and is said to offer a host of health benefits because it's packed with antioxidants and is a probiotic.

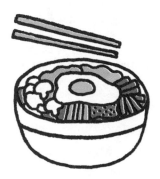

2. *Bibimbap.* A colorful and healthy dish with rice and an assortment of fresh veggies (thinly sliced carrots, roots, and spinach, to name a few) topped with a runny or fried egg. Mix the ingredients, and add a dollop of sesame oil and spicy red paste to taste. If you're on a Korean Air flight and bibimbap is one of the offerings, you can't go wrong.

3. *Haemul Pajeon.* This pancake-like dish is cut into slices and dipped

in soy sauce. It's made with a batter of egg and flour mixed with a variety of veggies like green onions and kimchi and seafood like clams, squid, and oysters. It's often enjoyed with *makgeolli,* a sweet rice wine.

4. *Mul Naengmyun.* While the words "cold noodles" might not get your blood pumping, this is a dish not to be ignored. Imagine buckwheat noodles in a cold beef broth topped with slices of cucumber, Korean pear, and a boiled egg, then seasoned with vinegar and *gyeoja* (a spicy mustard). It's typically served in the summer, often after eating generous portions of Korean BBQ.

5. *Samgyetang.* Traditionally enjoyed on the hottest day of the year—to "fight heat with heat"—*samgyetang* is a stewed whole young chicken stuffed with ginseng, garlic, rice, and scallions and served piping hot. It's believed that eating this dish three times a year brings optimal health benefits.

6. *Gamjatang.* This stew usually contains perilla leaves, which give it a lot of its delicious, rich flavor, and has a base of potatoes and pork spine. This dish is almost more delicious as leftovers: add rice and veggies to the soup reduction to make a scrumptious fried rice.

7. *Tteokguk. Tteokguk* is a beef broth soup garnished with slices of fried egg, pressed beef, and seaweed. It is traditionally eaten to celebrate the New Year and served with long oval strips of rice cake, which symbolize a long and healthy life.

8. *Samgyupsal.* What we've all been waiting for: Korean BBQ—Long strips of pork wrapped in lettuce leaves and coupled with grilled garlic slices, kimchi, soybean paste, and other *banchan*. The best

Korean BBQ is grilled over hot coals, not gas, and is frequently paired with soju.

9. *Tteokbokki.* A dish that manages to be both sweet and spicy. *Tteok-bokki* is sliced rice cakes smothered in red pepper paste and green onions. It's a fairly inexpensive dish that is best when eaten at street carts and paired with a cup of fishcake soup (called *oden*).

10. *Patbingsoo.* Dessert time! Made with ice shavings and traditionally topped with condensed milk, sweet red beans (*pat*), and rice cake (*tteok*), *patbingsoo* is crunchy and sweet. You can find many variations with fruit and ice cream served at cafés and restaurants.

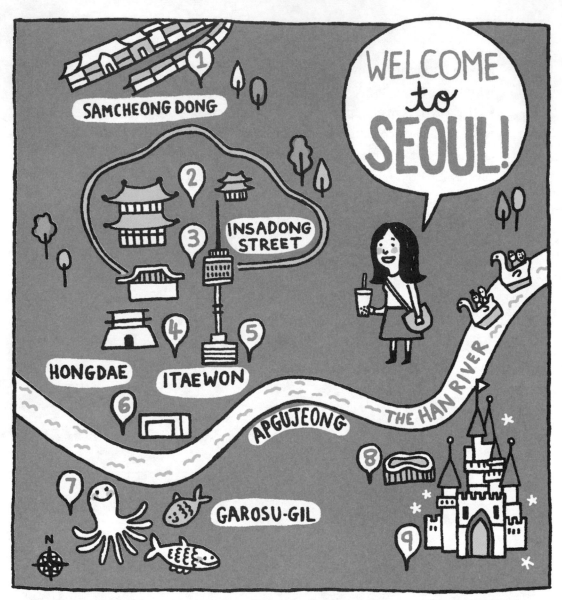

My Heart in Seoul:

Where to Eat, Drink, Shop, and Beautify

*H*ey-o!
 You probably never thought you'd make it this far in a skin-care book, so bravo you!

By now, I hope you've come to understand why "skin is in" in Korea, and that this mindset has inspired you to understand, learn about, and care for your own skin with the same level of enthusiasm.

And though this is the end of the book, it's obviously not the end of your skin-care education. There will always be more to research, new ingredients to get to know, and new innovations to try, but it's great to feel that you're the expert on your own skin and are hard at work getting it to be the healthiest it can be.

There's no such thing as perfect skin, but whether you're less flaky, have fewer break-outs, or look a bit dewier than when you started, well, those are all skin wins to be celebrated.

It's no secret that Seoul is a very special place to me, and Korea on the whole is a country that I care for unconditionally. My parents left Korea with no plans to return, but I think it was my fate to stumble upon this culture, find my calling, and embrace learning about the skin-care and beauty culture here. Through this book, I've been able to continue to explore Korea, and I hope that I've been able to share with you why it means so much to me. Maybe you now have your own bit of beauty wanderlust? That could be you, strolling the streets of Seoul, your arms laden with shopping bags full of sheet masks!

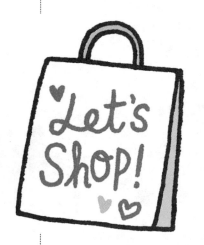

To be honest, living in Seoul was never on my bucket list. I actually plotted to make my big-girl move out to New York City (where I live now) right after college, but luck, chance, and fate led me on a detour through Seoul. It was about as far away as you could get from California, but once I was there, it didn't take me too long to realize that I'd never felt so at home. That "pit stop" turned into half a decade, and from those five years sprouted my passion for skin care and the opportunity to become an entrepreneur and the person I am today.

I want to share my love for Seoul because I know it's not a top destination for most tourists. Many just know of the city as a layover on the way to other Asian destinations, such as Bangkok or Beijing, but it's so much more than just an awesome airport (though trust me—the airport is really, truly awesome).

I think of Seoul as Asia's best-kept secret—one that needs to be shared.

I love the United States and consider myself very privileged to have grown up with the best of both worlds, but I truly think that—from the people to the food, the shopping, the nightlife, the culture, the energy, the service, and the history—there's no place like Korea. The pace of life is fast and furious in Seoul, and I love both what the city is now and what it's striving to be.

I hope that my love for Korea has inspired you to want to experience it for yourself someday. In fact, I hope this so much that I went ahead and put together an itinerary for you! Come on, you can never be too prepared!

Here's my mini-guide to Seoul—the full story on where I'd shop and eat and what I'd do if I had only seventy-two hours. Consider me a friend who's more than happy to show you around. Seoul moves fast, and stores and restaurants are constantly changing, so when you're planning your trip (yay!), use this chapter as a guide, but refer to SokoGlam.com for the latest updates.

xo— charlotte

Neighborhoods to Know

Myeong-dong (명동)

This legendary promenade is lined with more beauty shops than you ever imagined could be possible. Stand in the middle of an intersection and you'll see beauty stores every which way you turn. Outside the stores, brand ambassadors pass out samples to entice you in, and once you're in, they're ready to handle your beauty questions in multiple languages, too! I'd set aside three to four hours to explore all the beauty shops. I usually bring an extra-large bag or backpack (though I wish I had an extra set of arms) to carry all my goodies back home. It's great because in between your shopping, you can come up for air and snack at the food vendors lined up and down the main strip. Don't forget to sample the egg bread and, if you're adventurous, fried squid.

There are several big department stores (Lotte and Shinsegae, to name two well-known ones) within walking distance of Myeong-dong's main strip that can satisfy your appetite for more premium Korean beauty brands. In most department stores, you can find them nestled next to the international beauty brands on the ground floor.

How to get there: Myeong-dong Station (명동역)—Line 4, exit 6, or Euljiro 1-ga Station (을지로입구역)—Line 2, exit 6

Garosu-gil (가로수길)

Meaning "treelined street," Garosu-gil is a trendy area filled with boutiques, coffee shops, and restaurants. My favorite shop here is Jaju, which is stocked with Anthropologie-like housewares but at a fraction of the price, and Aland, which has a collection of indie fashion designer labels, and you'll be shocked at how affordable everything is (just don't be shocked at the minimal size runs, which is a frustrating fact about clothes in Korea). There is a Su:m37 brick-and-mortar here, too! Sadly, larger fast-fashion brands are starting to take over this very expensive strip of land and the biggest stores on the block are Forever 21 and H&M.

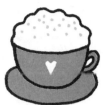

You won't go hungry or suffer caffeine withdrawal here, as coffee and pastry options are plentiful, with cafés on every corner. My personal favorite is Bloom and Goûté, which serves brunch all day and sells flowers, so it looks and smells amazing. I love exploring new coffee shops, and when I'm in Seoul, I'll take my laptop and pick a new one to work at every week.

This hood is also where you'll find me brunching with a bunch of girl-friends, and I definitely try to dress my best when I come out to Garosugil. The people watching is amazing, and you'll see some of the trendiest fashionistas in the world here.

How to get there: Sinsa Station (신사역)—Line 3, exit 8 (ten-minute walk)

Hongdae (홍대)

Hongdae is known for its young, artsy crowd and its vibrant nightlife, which is spillover from nearby Hongik University, one of Korea's popular universities. Lots of beauty brand shops are clustered here, and inexpensive nail salons are plentiful! If you're in the mood to shop clothing,

Stylenanda (en.stylenanda.com) is one of my favorite boutiques. Hongdae really comes alive at night, though, when people fill the streets en route to and from its many bars and clubs. This is a great spot for drinking soju and eating *anju*, which is a word to describe snacks served with alcoholic beverages, only better. Many spots here actually won't let you order alcohol without *anju*, so just think of it as if they're looking out for you.

How to get there: Hongik University Station (홍대입구역)—Line 2, exit 9, or Sangsu Station (상수역)—Line 6, exit 1

Itaewon (이태원)

Dave and I spent many nights in Itaewon, as it's right next to the U.S. Army base where he was stationed. It was once known primarily for its appeal to U.S. service members and a large expat community, but it's now enjoyed by both Koreans and non-Koreans alike. It has a vibrant nightlife, with lots of international restaurants and many tiny, winding alleys that are home to eclectic bars and lounges. If you want non-Korean food options like tacos (Vatos Urban Tacos, vatoskorea.com) or pulled pork sandwiches (Linus' Bama Style Barbecue), you'll likely find it here, and you won't be disappointed. Come Friday and Saturday nights (and super early Sunday mornings), this is where you can find me.

During daylight hours, I'll be at my favorite shoe boutique, Chaussure Lapin (chaussurelapin.com), which makes custom shoes if you give them about a week. Guys, if you go to Hamilton Shirts (hs76.com), you can get some really affordable and sharp custom shirts and suits made within a week.

How to get there: Itaewon Station (이태원역)—Line 6, any exit

Samcheong-dong (삼청동)

This neighborhood is the perfect intersection of old meets new. There are tons of dessert and coffee shops, art galleries, and boutiques to browse through, all hidden down small, curving streets and in buildings that nod to traditional Korean architecture and housing. It seems as if there's always a new store or restaurant to check out in Samcheong-dong, so no visit is ever the same. I love walking through here on a quiet Sunday morning. There are a few popular *mat jib*s serving classic Korean comfort foods like *tteokbokki* (spicy rice cake), and it's only a ten-minute walk from the arts district, Insa-dong, where there are many traditional teahouses and even more art galleries. Insa-dong is a bit too touristy for my taste, so I don't spend too much time there, but if it's your first time in Seoul, it's definitely worth strolling through.

> *How to get to Samcheong-dong: Anguk Station (안국역)—Line 3, exit 1*
> *How to get to Insa-dong: Anguk Station (안국역)—Line 3, exit 6*

Gwangjang Market (광장시장)

Gwangjang Market is one of the oldest outdoor markets in South Korea, and when I'm in the mood to experience something more traditional, it's hard to beat going here and chowing down on some classic Korean comfort food. There are also beautiful linens, bedding, and even traditional dresses for sale here.

It seems as if a night market like this would always be overrun with tourists, but locals make up the bulk of the crowd here, which makes me love it even more. Outdoor food stalls open at 9 A.M. and go until 11 P.M. If you're a foodie like me and like to eat your way through cities, come here for the mung bean pancake (*bindaetteok*, 빈대떡), the steak tartare (*yukhoe*, 육회), or the seaweed rice rolls (*kimbap*, 김밥), which are so addictive that they're often called "crack kimbap."

How to get there: Jongno 5-ga Station (종로5가역)—Line 1, exit 8, or Euljiro 4-ga Station (을지로4가역)—Line 2, Line 5, exit 4

You've Found the Restaurant— Now What? How to Order

Sitting down at a restaurant in Seoul can be a bit overwhelming if you don't speak the language, but once you get the lay of the land and how to order, I wouldn't be surprised if Korean service ruins you for all other dining experiences.

When you sit down, look for a button at the edge of the table. When you're ready to order, press it to alert your server. Most traditional Korean restaurants have this button, and it is so much more efficient than trying

#SOKOSecret A friendly way to address female servers is by calling them *unni*, which means "older sister," or *emo*, which means "auntie," no matter if you're older or younger. For men, the standard *yeogiyo* is sufficient.

to wave somebody down. If there's no button, feel free to call your server if you want their attention by saying loudly and firmly, *"Yeogiyo!"* It means "excuse me, I need some attention over here" and it's normal to call them over like that!

For the essentials, you don't even need your server! Most utensils, carafes of water, napkins, and cups will be readily available at your table (or tucked away inside a drawer of the table, so check there if not on top). Distribute utensils to all the guests to place on top of napkins and pour water for your neighbors.

> #SoKoSecret: Just a warning: If you provide utensils and pour water for only yourself, it can be perceived as pretty selfish, so always, always serve others before you serve yourself.

There's a lot of respect shown at mealtimes. Don't start eating until the eldest person at the table does. Also, when receiving anything (a soju shot or even a cup of water) make it a habit to receive with both hands. It seems like a small thing, but it speaks volumes if you show that simple sign of respect.

When you want to pay your bill, just look for the check at the table (it's probably already tallied up and ready to be taken to the counter at the entrance of the restaurant). Paying on your way out is super efficient and eliminates any back-and-forth with your waiter. Also, chances are there's a handy mirror on your way out, which makes it convenient to do a quick teeth check for unwanted food wedgies (see, Korean restaurants really do think of everything!).

Despite the superfast, phenomenal service (sometimes at a BBQ, a server will even stand over your table grilling and cutting your meat for most of the meal, though you can do it yourself if you're comfortable), tipping is not required—at all! There's no tip line available on a credit card slip. If you do tip, someone might chase you out and say you left too much cash on the table. That being said, I've tipped everyone from my hair stylist to cab-drivers, and though they are usually surprised, its always been much appreciated.

Shopping Tips

· ·

- Skip the luxury brands or anything you can buy at home. Korea has a luxury tax, which means they'll be more expensive here. Most of these luxury brands live in Korea's largest department stores, but I'd still check out Hyundai Department Store if I were you just because there's so much more than what you'd experience at a typical Western department store. It has an amazing food court and bakery section and even a high-end grocery store built in. Also, as mentioned before, you can buy more prestige brand Korean beauty products like Sulwhasoo and O HUI here.
- Bring cash so you can exchange your currency to Korean won (KRW) at the airport. Most ATMs won't let you withdraw from a credit or debit card. You'll want cash for all the cool street vendors selling everything from the latest (and prettiest) cell phone cases to hair accessories and socks. Can you ever have enough cute socks? No, you cannot! A lot of boutiques also give you discounts from 5 to 10 percent if you pay with cash. Also, don't be scared to haggle! It's not

uncommon for sellers to knock off 1,000 to 2,000 KRW (equivalent to a buck or two) from the initial price.

• If you want strictly Korean-made fashion, there are fashion malls like Doota and Migliore located in Dongdaemun. While Korea is

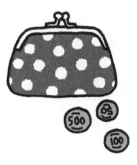

famous for its fashion district in Dongdaemun, especially for its night market, which opens at 9 P.M., just be warned it's not as cheap as you might expect. Sometimes it's better to shop near women's universities such as Ewha Womans University, where you'll find affordable Korean threads. Because Korean clothing is distributed to many vendors, you may find the same exact dress in Garosu-gil (but for a premium price).

• If you're looking for bargains, you can go shopping underground by a major subway station such as the Express Bus Terminal Station (고속터미널역), Gangnam Station (강남역), and Jamsil Station (잠실역). Underground malls showcase tons of inexpensive fashion boutiques and cosmetic brands and also have lots of snack stands selling tasty treats if you get hungry from all the shopping.

• Sometimes clothing stores won't allow you to try on blouses, sweaters, or dresses that aren't button-down. This is so customers won't stain clothes with makeup. If this happens to you, don't be offended—it's just store policy.

My Favorite Korean Spas

Since no trip to Seoul would be complete without a trip to the *jimjilbang,* here are a few to check out.

Dragon Hill Spa and Resort

I used to live near this Korean spa, so I would come here all the time. It's one of the largest spas in Seoul and it has *all* the bells and whistles—it's the Vegas of Korean spas. The dry saunas include a charcoal kiln sauna, a pine tree sauna, a red clay sauna, a crystal sun salt room, and a meditation room, and wet saunas include a natural bedrock seawater bath, Korean ginseng bath, Hinoki tub . . . I could go on, but you get the idea! There's even a game room and an outdoor pool, and you can also get treatments like traditional body scrubs, facials, and massages. At times it can be too crowded with tourists, but many locals still make frequent visits.

How to get there: Sinyongsan Station (신용산역)—Line 4, exit 4
www.dragonhillspa.co.kr

Spa Lei

I like this Korean spa because it's female only, and it seems more intimate (there are fewer families, so it's slightly less chaotic) and laid-back compared with Dragon Hill Spa. You can sit in a sagebrush tub or an open-air hot tub, take a half-body bath for circulation (which works off the principle that the head should be cool and the feet should be warm), and partake in a host of other tubs, treatments, and saunas.

How to get there: Sinsa Station (신사역)—Line 3, exit 5
www.spalei.co.kr

Nail Shops: Full-Service Salons for Nails, Waxing, and Eyelash Extensions

Every neighborhood has tons of nail shops; you just need to keep your eyes peeled as you explore Seoul. And I kid you not, any nail shop you enter, you're going to have pretty great service and really skilled designers, so you don't need to worry if you're going to a popular chain or not. Depending on what neighborhood you go to, the cost can fluctuate. For example, near college campuses like Ewha Womans University, the nail shops will be a little smaller and dingier, but the price will be low compared with getting your nails done in an upscale neighborhood like Cheongdam-dong.

Keep in mind nail shops offer eyelash extensions and waxing services as well! Eyelash extensions are extremely popular in Korea because it looks so natural and you can avoid wearing mascara every day. Waxing is still not a huge thing in Korea, but it is getting more popular. For your one-stop shop for beautification, check out these shops below.

Witch Nails

I was drawn to this nail shop because of its awesome name. If you come here, make it worth your while and do something extremely funky and creative! Look through the gallery of nail art options, or arm yourself with photos to show the designers exactly what you want, as they can likely replicate it and then some. Witch Nails offers eyelash extensions and waxing services as well. If you can, try calling in advance to make reservations because it can get pretty booked!

How to get there: Sinsa Station (신사역)—Line 3, exit 8 (ten-minute walk to Garosu-gil, 2nd floor)

http://blog.naver.com/witch_nail

Coco Lounge

I love this beauty shop because it does everything at a reasonable price and has an English-speaking staff, since it is located in Itaewon and is a frequent stop for expats. Coco Lounge provides full wax services, manis, pedis, laser hair removal, massages, and even (gasp—not that you would ever do it) tanning!

How to get there: Itaewon Station (이태원역)—Line 6, any exit

www.facebook.com/cocoloungekorea

Facials

Affordable facials are plentiful in Seoul, especially if you buy a facial package, which is usually sold in packs of ten treatments for around 200,000

KRW (which works out to less than 20 USD per facial). If you're just visiting Seoul, you can still partake in single treatments for around 30,000–40,000 KRW (approximately 30–40 USD). I frequented a very affordable and popular chain that many locals go to called MI-PL (www.mipl.co.kr). In a typical facial, expect a lot of shoulder and chest(!) massages to be included in the treatment.

For a more luxurious spa experience, check out the spa services available at major hotels such as the Shilla or the Banyan Tree Club and Spa. If you want to get a brand-specific spa service, I recommend checking out the signature green tea spa treatments at the Amore Spa, located in the Lotte department store (*Euljiro 1-ga Station—Line 2, exit 7*), and for herbal facial treatments, go to Hanyul Jeong Spa (*Myeong-dong Station—Line 4, exit 6*).

Hair Salons

Franck Provost

Although the salon is technically a French brand, all the stylists are Korean and they never disappoint. I stumbled upon this hair salon and have never looked back. It's a very cozy yet chic salon that's never too crowded, and I can always pop in even without an appointment. When a coloring session ran long, they made me toast, tea, and a cappuccino. I've received amazing massages, too, all free of charge.

How to get there: Sinsa Station (신사역)—Line 3, exit 8 (2/F Sinsa-dong Gangnam-gu)

Juno Hair

Juno Hair is a major chain, so you can find this hair salon in most neighborhoods. I go here whenever I need a quick blowout or trim. They're very efficient so you're in and then you're out. They don't skimp on the service here either—they give amazing head massages when shampooing. A blowout is no more than 20,000 KRW (less than 20 USD), and no tip!

How to get there: Gangnam Station (강남역)—Line 2, exit 11 (3/F Jaeyeong Building Gangnam-gu)

www.junohair.com

Jenny House

If you want to experience a full-service, upscale Korean salon, Jenny House will be your jam. My visit was on a Saturday and it was packed with brides and grooms prepping for their engagement photos or their wedding, but the place ran like a well-oiled machine. If you want the latest in hair, makeup, and nail art, you've come to the right place. Plus, you might spot a Korean celebrity or two!

How to get there: Apgujeong Rodeo Station (압구정로데오역)—Bundang Line, exit 2 (Jenny House Primo)

www.jennyhouse.co.kr

Dermatologists

. . . .

Arumdaun Nara Beauty Clinic

There are tons of dermatologists and clinics in Seoul, but if you're going to visit one you should probably find one that offers services in English, since communication will be key to receiving the proper treatment. Arumdaun Nara is a popular clinic I've been to, and it's conveniently located right by Gangnam Station (강남역). Like any dermatologist clinic in Korea, it offers a full list of treatments: facials, laser treatments for wrinkles, procedures for acne scarring, even Botox and dermal fillers. There are more than eight dermatologists and a handful of estheticians in the clinic to also make it a one-stop shop for your specific skin-care needs.

How to get there: Gangnam Station (강남역)—Line 2, exit 2 (5/F Yeoksam-dong Gangnam-gu)

http://anacli.co.kr/english/01intro/intro01.asp

The Reason We're All Here: Beauty Shopping!

. . . .

Since you're going to want to pick up as much as you can for yourself, your besties, and your mom, you'll want to know what brands and products to look out for and why. The largest cosmetic company in Korea is Amore-Pacific, and it has got a ton of brands under its belt, such as Innisfree, Etude

House, Laneige, IOPE, and Sulwhasoo. The next largest cosmetic company is LG Household & Health Care (LG H&H), and it's the maker of Su:m37, O HUI, The Faceshop, Belif, and Beyond. In addition to these two power-houses, there are a ton of great, quality brands that are not under these umbrellas, and I encourage you to explore new brands as much as you can!

The list below has some of my favorite brands and their superstar products. Keep in mind that Korean brands renew their product names, packaging, and lines frequently, so brands and products mentioned below may be reincarnated into something else or discontinued. Check out SokoGlam .com for the latest.

AmorePacific

Green tea, bamboo sap, and red ginseng are the core Asian botanicals that AmorePacific formulates its products with. A premium brand with luxurious packaging, I can't get enough of its bestsellers: the Treatment Enzyme Peel and the Color Control Cushion Compact.

www.us.amorepacific.com

Banila Co.

Banila Co. is an urban brand with a youthful yet sophisticated vibe—think glowing pink-and-white stores that look like they came straight from the future. Although it's famous for its CC cream (the first brand to produce it in Korea), it also has a wide array of popular products that appeals to consumers in markets outside of Korea. My all-time favorite oil-based cleanser, the Banila Co. Clean It Zero cleansing balm, is also its best seller, and its newly launched VV line (named for the inclusion of "vitalizing serum" in its formulations) is one of the hottest new products on the market.

www.banilaco.com

Belif

Walk into Belif and you'll feel like you're in a European apothecary, which is a nod to the brand's traditional herbal formulas combined with modern cosmetic science. A cult favorite is the Aqua Bomb, a cream that offers intense hydration and moisture (even for oily skin types, thanks to its gel-like consistency). Even though you can get Belif products at Sephora, it's worth a visit in Seoul because Belif does not have any independent brick-and-mortar stores in the United States—yet.

www.belifcosmetic.com

Chosungah

I'm a big fan of the makeup artist Cho Sung Ah's design and aesthetic, in both her makeup and skin-care lines. Chosungah's punchy, loud colors and unique packaging are an instant pick-me-up to your beauty routine. The Raw Black Bubble cleanser, which functions as both a cleanser and a mask, was a hit in Korea and I completely understand why.

www.chosungah22.com

Clio

To me, this is Korea's answer to MAC. Clio is focused on professional-grade color cosmetics from foundation to matte lipsticks. It's also home to my holy grail product: the Waterproof Pen Liner. Stock up on Clio's long-lasting, vibrant lip stains and eyeliners to channel that Kpop look back home.

www.clubcliousa.com

Neogen Dermalogy

Neogen Dermalogy can be found throughout Korea and in major cities in Asia, and several K-beauty trends were jump-started by its one-of-a-kind packaging, formulas, and products. The Neogen Dermalogy Real Fresh Foam cleanser contains real cranberries or green tea in the bottle and is one of the bestsellers at Olive Young (a multi-brand beauty store you'll see everywhere). The latest buzzworthy product is its Bio Peel Gauze Peeling Wine, which comes with unique three-layer pads for exfoliation.

www.neogenderma.com

Etude House

Entering this shop will feel as if you just entered a real human-size dollhouse filled from top to bottom with the cutest beauty products! Though it may feel kitschy at first, don't underestimate the brand—after all, Etude House is a child company of cosmetics giant AmorePacific. Some of my favorite skin-care products and lippies are from this store, such as the Moistfull Collagen line and the My Jelly Lips-Talk lippies.

www.etudehouse.com

The Faceshop

You might be familiar with the name and the store, as The Faceshop made a splash in the early 2000s as one of the first major K-beauty brands to set up shop in the United States. Some of the best eyebrow pencils and cleansing oils I've used have come from its ridiculously affordable selection of quality goods.

www.international.thefaceshop.com

Goodal

Goodal, a sister brand of Clio, prides itself in using fermentation as the core of its formulas. Its light, gel-like formulas are great for acne-prone skin, especially its Super Seed Oil Plus line, which includes green tea extract, licorice root extract, and niacinamide to help even skin tone, improve skin's elasticity, and reduce oil production.

www.goodal.co.kr

Innisfree

Koreans and tourists alike go gaga for this brand because of the clean packaging and the use of natural ingredients derived from Jeju Island. Reasonably priced and another knockout brand from AmorePacific, I have so many Innisfree favorites I can't possibly list them all. For starters, try its Olive Oil Real Cleansing Tissue, Olive Real Cleansing Oil, No-Sebum Mineral Powder, and Jeju Volcanic Pore Clay Mask.

www.innisfreeworld.com

IOPE

IOPE focuses on fusing enriched herbal extracts with the latest in skin-care technology, which has resulted in some of the most cutting-edge products on the market, like the IOPE Air Cushion! An AmorePacific brand, it was the first to develop the innovative cushion compact. Since then, its innovation has spawned many copycats from Korean to global brands alike, but if you want to experience the OG cushion compact (and in my opinion still the best in formula and sponge technology), don't accept any substitutes.

www.iope.com

It's Skin

It's Skin made its mark in the Korean cosmetic beauty scene with its snail mucin products, which are wildly popular. If you're looking to reduce acne scarring through the power of snail mucin extract, try the Prestige Crème Ginseng de Escargot line.

www.itsskin.com/eng/index.asp

Laneige

This brand places its focus on using water science to deeply hydrate the skin and protect it from environmental stressors. I've used Laneige's Water Sleeping Mask for years, and I'm pleased to see that it continues to be a bestseller, even though many sleeping masks have entered the market since. Also it would be worthwhile to check out its BB cushion at Target, because there are more shade variations for the U.S. market than there are in Korea.

www.us.laneige.com

Manefit

This brand is a secret gem, as its sheet masks are made from one of Korea's top mask manufacturers, so you get extremely high-quality products without paying for the brand name. Check out its Bling Bling Hydrogel Mask and its sister brand, Ultru, for hydration, brightening, and dewy results.

Missha

Missha is well known internationally for several of its star products: M Perfect Cover BB cream, Time Revolution First Treatment Essence, and Time Revolution Night Repair Science Activator Ampoule. I personally love how the brand focuses on providing high-quality skin-care products without the luxury price tag. The Time Revolution essence and ampoule are dupes of more expensive luxury-brand products, which makes it easier on the wallet while delivering very comparable results.

www.misshaus.com

O HUI

O HUI is a premium line that's found in department stores like Hyundai. It's most known for using science to enhance and protect the functionality of the skin through sensitive skin formulas. I really enjoy the lightweight feel of most of its products and its focus on hydration to keep skin healthy, elastic, and dewy. If you want to splurge, the First Cell Revolution Essence is one of my favorite essences.

www.ohui.co.kr

RE:P

RE:P is an environmentally conscious brand that formulates their products with organically grown ingredients and without parabens, mineral oil, or animal byproducts. Their packaging is also made with 100 percent de-inked post-consumer waste and printed with soy ink. For the optimal organic experience, try their Organic Cotton Treatment Toning pad or their Fresh Mask with Real Calming Herb.

Skinfood

Feed your skin with the same nutritious food you would feed your body. From avocados and eggplants to egg whites and tomatoes, Skinfood believes in using the nutrients derived from food to supplement and protect your skin. Packaging that is both whimsical and functional (and affordable), my personal favorites include the Black Sugar Mask Wash Off and the Avocado Leave-In Fluid as a conditioner for hair.

www.eng.theskinfood.com

Son & Park

Son & Park is a brand created by two leading Korean makeup artists, Son Dae Sik and Park Tae Yun. Friends since high school, they developed a genuine flair for colors and became masters at creating natural and flawless looks. Son Dae Sik is also the official makeup artist for Jeon Ji Hyun, arguably one of the most famous actresses in Korea currently. Son & Park's Skin Fit Foundation flies off the shelves because it provides natural coverage and has an essence base formulated in the middle of the stick. I also covet their Beauty Water, a smart toner and exfoliator in one.

www.sonandpark.com

Su:m37

Su:m37 is a premium beauty brand in Korea that specializes in naturally fermented skin-care products. "Su:m" represents the Korean word for "respiration" and "37" signifies the optimal temperature for the fermentation process. If I had to choose two of my favorites products, they would be the Miracle Rose Cleansing Stick and the Water-full Timeless Moisturizing Cream.

www.su-m37.com/english

Sulwhasoo

Sulwhasoo is a high-end luxury skin-care brand that formulates its products using medicinal herbs (such as ginseng and white lily) to balance the inner energies of the skin using traditional Korean methods. If you're into holistic skin care, pick up its star product: the Concentrated Ginseng Renewing Cream. My personal favorite is the Essential Renewing Eye Cream.

www.us.sulwhasoo.com

Swagger

One of the most popular men's lifestyle brands, Swagger has a wide selection of essential skin-care and hair products. As the name would suggest, the packaging is sleek and perfect for the male urban dweller. Dave uses the Hair Slammer Pomade, which you can pick up at the nearest Olive Young.

www.swagger.kr

Tony Moly

Tony Moly initially stood out for its fun, adorable packaging, which started with sweet-smelling hand creams shaped like animals and pieces of fruit, and its youthful appeal keeps customers coming back. The brand is known for its BCDation foundation and its sheer and moisturizing Petite Bunny Gloss Bars.

www.tonymolyus.com

3CE

This edgy cosmetic brand, launched by Korea's rising fashion brand StyleNanda, is known for its long-lasting formulas and the intensity of its modern colors. It's hard not to splurge on their Lip Crayons and Highlight Beam, not to mention their fun nail art accessories.

www.en.stylenanda.com

Too Cool for School

This is not your typical K-beauty brand. Too Cool for School doesn't even use Korean models to promote its brand because its goods are already coveted worldwide for both their quality and whimsical, innovative packaging. It'll be hard to leave Too Cool's intricately decorated shop without taking home something from its Dinoplatz line. Your next challenge will be to actually use the product—the packaging is so good that you'll experience a tiny pang of regret at breaking the seal and opening it.

www.toocoolforschool.com

Multi-Brand Shops

Olive Young, Watsons, and Belport are essentially upscale beauty drugstores. They carry a wide array of midpriced brands (both Korean and international). There are tons of gems to be found there, so they are definitely worth a gander.

The Basic Essentials

• •

Subway and Taxi: How to Get Around

- Whenever and wherever you can, take the subway! It's awesome, with climate-controlled seats, air-conditioning, and LCD screens to display train arrival times. Subways in Seoul are generally clean and run very frequently (which can be a shock if you're used to the New York subway system!). It can get super crowded during rush hour, and most lines stop running around midnight, so if you take the subway on a night out, plan to have an alternative way of getting home.

- Taxis in Seoul are relatively inexpensive and very plentiful (the starting base fare is less than 3 USD, and they take both credit cards and cash). You know if the taxi is available if the LED sign on the windshield is red and shows the characters 빈차, which means "empty car." The characters 예약, mean "reserved." You know that the taxi is not available when the LED characters are turned off. For safety reasons, only the right passenger door can be opened to get in and out. The left door is usually locked from the inside. Stay off the roads during rush hour—Seoul traffic can be pretty painful, so stick to the subway when you can.

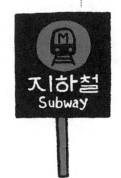

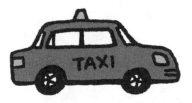

This can be annoying for tourists, but destinations are not easily reached via street addresses. Most of the time you have to go by popular landmarks, major intersections, or even subway stops. If you're having trouble communicating with your taxi driver (some do speak and understand English, but don't assume they will!), having a smartphone would be handy so you can show him what landmark or area you're trying to get to.

Free Wi-Fi—It's Everywhere!

Wi-Fi is readily available literally everywhere, from coffee shops that don't mind if you camp out and work for hours to public areas like Gangnam Station. If you need something more reliable, you can rent a portable Wi-Fi router at the airport when you land. It'll cost you about 8 USD a day and works pretty well. Use messaging apps to communicate with your friends so you can avoid data roaming charges.

Korean Beauty Shopping at Home!

Soko Glam

Aka my baby, Soko Glam (short for South Korean Glam) is a Korean beauty and lifestyle e-shop. I personally test all products and curate only the ones I love and think you'll love, too. My passion is to help people of all ages better understand their skin so that they can look and feel their best, while they discover the wonderful world of Korean beauty products.

www.sokoglam.com

The Klog

For more skin care tips and in-depth product reviews about the innovative and fascinating world of Korea—you're in luck! I'm also the editor-in-chief of The Klog, a Korean beauty content site that is your inside source on beauty trends, culture vibes, and a peek into the world of Korean women and men. So it's more than just moisturizer. It's an inside look at the world we love, and The Klog has the stories.

www.theklog.co

Urban Outfitters

Urban Outfitters carries select items from several Korean brands, from Clio to Skinfood.

www.urbanoutfitters.com

Sephora

Sephora carries select products from AmorePacific, Too Cool for School, Dr.Jart+, Belif, and Tony Moly.

www.sephora.com

Target

Target carries select products from the brand Laneige.

www.target.com

Amazon

Through Amazon you can search for and buy a wide assortment of Korean beauty products. Just know that some of the products are coming directly from Korea, so you may have to wait longer than the standard three to five business days.

www.amazon.com

Brand Shops

Several Korean beauty brands currently have brick-and-mortar stores in major metropolitan areas in the United States, including Tony Moly, Skinfood, Aritaum (a shop selling AmorePacific brands), Clio, The Faceshop, Missha, and Nature Republic. Also, more of these brands are expanding their e-commerce offerings for customers in the United States, but, depending on the brand, their products could be shipping from Korea, so you may have to deal with a longer wait than with U.S.-based e-shops.

In cities like New York and Los Angeles, which have large Koreatowns, you can often find random assortments of products in Korean cosmetics shops. These stores are usually a hodgepodge of brands and items and won't be the place to go for expert advice, but you can usually pick up an inexpensive sheet mask, nail polish, or lipstick to try out. Just Yelp "Korean cosmetics" and prepare yourself for an adventure.

SKIN STORIES: Jenn Im

DIGITAL INFLUENCER AND VLOGGER OF *CLOTHES ENCOUNTERS*

The shopping experience in Seoul is unlike that in any other city I've visited. On my recent trip to Seoul, I went back home with a ton of beauty products and clothing. My favorite area to shop for clothes was probably Hongdae—I really loved how there was a store on every corner. I was blown away by the reasonable prices and the quality of the pieces. Most clothing items were lined, and there's a heavy attention to detail in the structure of clothing made in Korea. Right now, I'm still really inspired by the brand Stylenanda. From the clothing to the makeup, they have such a fresh and cute appeal.

I also love people watching in Seoul. I noticed the makeup trends are quite subtle and tend toward a more innocent look. My favorite trends are the straight brow and the lip gradient. When I shop for beauty, I look for cushion compacts because they apply so seamlessly. I love how smooth and blended my skin looks afterward. I don't carry too much makeup with me, because I don't like a heavy purse. I really carry only a lip balm, hand cream, and one statement lip color. My lip color of choice is usually a vibrant coral that gives me a quick "oomph" factor if I'm needing one.

I make it a point to stop by Seoul every few years because the city changes so fast and there is always much to explore.

Acknowledgments

I've been blessed with so much that I secretly worry I've used up all the luck and love that one can possibly be granted in a lifetime. This book was just another gift from God, and it wouldn't have been possible had I not been surrounded by so many talented and genuine people. Words cannot express my gratitude, but I will try my best here.

First, I'd like to thank my best friend, husband, and Soko Glam co-founder, David Cho, who has supported my dream and vision since day one and has worked tirelessly to make the company what it is today. Without you, Soko Glam would have only been a "what if." Thanks for being there to give me pep talks whenever I needed one and for driving Soko Glam forward with the leadership you were born with. I'm so glad we're in this together.

Hong Sung-il Sangmoonim, there are few people in this world like you and I'm glad you were the one who walked into the meeting room my first day at Samsung. From the depths of my heart, thank you for your wisdom and for believing in me.

To Catherine Cho and Erin Niumata, for reading my words and seeing that I had a book in me—and then making the process so enjoyable! For all of this and more, I am eternally grateful.

Thank you to Jessamine Chen, for telling me to dream big when I needed to hear it, and to Jodi Kantor, who set me on the right path.

To Cassie Jones, my editor at HarperCollins—I knew from the moment I met you that the book would be in good hands with you. Needless to say, you exceeded my expectations a hundred times over.

To Gemma Correll, the most clever illustrator and artist around. The world needs more artists like you. Thank you for going above and beyond every time—your illustrations made the book better than I had even imagined.

To my dream editor, Kate Williams. Thank you for lending your wit, sass, and eloquence and for being by my side every step of the way. When you gave me the green light, I pinched myself because it was too good to be true. I simply couldn't have done it without you.

To all the people who were kind enough to share their experiences through such insightful interviews: Young Ah Kim, Soo Joo Park, India-Jewel Jackson, Kim Ju Won, Yeon-seo Oh, Paul Kang, Son Dae Sik, and Jenn Im.

To the other key people who helped make this book possible: Bradley Horowitz, Brian Lee, Don Kim, Yoo Hye Yun, Janet Kim, Lee Sang-Jun, Shawn Kim, Kim Chung Kyung, Lee Jung Won, and Lee Hee-Kyeong.

It's with a thankful heart that I mention the friends who have supported me along the way, especially when Soko Glam was just a dinky website and an apartment filled with Korean beauty products: Vickie Chang, Christine Chen, Jackie Chen, Annie Cheng, James Cho, Hellen Choo, Jeffrey Chou,

Emily Cleghorn, CEO Han Ho Lee, Yun Ah Lee, Jay Koo, Angie Lee, Annie Tomlin, Slava Druker, Stephanie Sherline, David Moretti, Ryan Browne, Tiffany J. Davis, Sheryll Donerson, Bob Dorf, Anne-Marie Guarnieri, Sara Hayden, Carolyn Hsu, Tae Jo, Robert Joe, Don Kim, Tay Kim, Erika Kindsfather, Helen Koo, Alvin Lee, Teresa Lu, Coco Park, Caitlin Petrecik, Phillip Picardi, Mark and Myoung-bin Ro, Yaeri Song, Kerry Thompson, Danny Tomita, Driely Vieria, Juliana Wang, Cheryl Wischhover, Annie Won, Diana Xiao, and Kim Yoon-jin. Of course, I can't forget my colleagues at Samsung, who made me feel right at home, and Dave and I can't forget all our friends from Columbia Business School.

As expressed in my dedication and throughout the book, I thank my father, Lee Ki Chul, and mother, Lee Sang Ran, both of whom taught me the meaning of hard work and sacrifice. Their unconditional love granted me the freedom to pursue my dreams and experience more than I could have ever imagined in both the United States and Korea. To my mother-in-law, Nancy Cho, who taught Dave about skin care at an early age and was our biggest supporter (and customer). To my unni, Michelle Yoon, who is truly beautiful inside and out—thank you for letting me tag along to all those Kpop concerts in the 1990s. To my *dongsaeng,* Brian Lee, who is the most honest and considerate man I know. Special thanks to Kim Yong Bae and Lee Myung Ok and family, who showed me *jeong* and treated me as their own. Kim Min Young, thanks for sharing your world and always wanting the best for me.

My deepest thanks to our Soko Glam customers—for sharing our passion for Korean beauty and for making *all* of this possible. Lastly, to South Korea and America, for giving me the opportunity and the inspiration to build something out of nothing.

Index

hyperpigmentation, 51, 52
hypoallergenic products, 124–25
Hyun, Jeon Ji, 155

I

ice igloo, 58
Im, Jenn, 202–3
Innisfree, 193
IOPE, 193–94
IOPE Air Cushion XP, 145–46
Italy towels, 49, 56
It's Skin, 194

J

Jackson, India-Jewel, 62–63
jade sauna, 58
jeong, 61–62
jimjilbang, 52–58
jojoba beads, 49

K

Kang, Paul, 132–33
Kdramas, 10, 148, 155
Kim, Young Ah, 26–27
kojic acid, 130
Korean Air flight attendants, 141–42

Korean beauty industry
affordable products in, 23–24, 128
beauty shopping at home, 200–202
competition in, 19–20, 26, 127
focus on health, 132–33, 157–59
high-quality products, 127–29
innovation in, 20, 128
largest cosmetic company, 189–90
multipurpose products, 115
new and powerful ingredients, 128–29
product packaging, 20–21, 26, 129
rise in product popularity, 18–19
"whitening" products, 23
Korean culture, 5–13, 15–16, 58–62, 136–38
Korean dishes, 169–71
Korean skin care
applying the products, 22
for children, 21–22
culture of, 5–13, 15–16
focus on healthy skin, 21
holistic nature of, 19
ideal of dewy skin, 22–23

motivation for, 102
number of products used, 22
as part of total health, 102–3
proven results from, 25–26
purpose behind each product, 22
treatments in, 70
trial-and-error process, 24
Korean spas
all-ages nature of, 52–53, 60
checking in, 53
dry saunas, 58
family rooms, 57
heated floors, 57
nudity, 53, 54
in Seoul, 184–85
showers, 53–54
treatments and body scrubs, 55–56
wet rooms, 54–55

L

lactic acid, 50–51, 130
Laneige, 194
laser treatments, 113
lash extensions, 153, 185
lifestyle, healthy, 157–69
lines, fine, 47, 68, 71, 109
lipids, 72

lip tint, 148–49, 154
loofahs, 47
lotions, 73

M

makeup
  removing, 31, 34–35,
    104–5
  routines, 133
  SPF, 95, 98
mandelic acid, 131
Manefit, 194
manufacturing dates, 126
mascara, 34–35, 104–5
massages, 55
metalloproteinases,
  87–88
McElligott, Bill, 93
melanin, 96
men, 123–24, 139–40
microfiber sheet masks,
  75, 79
Missha, 195
moisturizers
  after exfoliating, 51
  after shower, 41
  on damp face, 69
  importance of, 68
  for no-makeup look, 152
  in ten-step routine,
    111–12
  treatments before,
    70–71
  types of, 72–79

moles, 98
mugwort tea pool, 55
Multi-Brand Shops, 198
*My Love from Another
  Star*, 148, 155

N

nail shops, 185–86
Neogen Dermalogy, 192
niacinamide, 130
nicotine, 166
no makeup look
  for flight attendants,
    141–42
  instructions for, 151–55
  products for, 143–51

O

oatmeal, 49
Obama, Barack, 162
officetel, 59
Oh, Yeon-seo, 115
O HUI, 195
oil cleansers, 35–38,
  104–5
oral hygiene, 151

P

papain, 50
Park, Soo Joo, 44
PA system, 91

period-after-opening
  (PAO) symbol, 126
pH, 39–43
pimples, 31, 49, 121
plastic surgery, 138–39
pollution, 31, 32–33
pools, 55
pores, 31, 73, 106, 120
premarital sex, 163

R

red raspberry extract,
  131
"refreshers," 42, 107
RE:P, 195
restaurants, 180–82
retinol, 51, 71, 98
rosacea, 40, 88
rotating brush, 50

S

saccharomyces ferment
  filtrate, 131
salicylic acid, 51, 106,
  121, 130
salt sauna, 58
Samsung, 164
sebum, 31, 35, 50
selcas, 77
Seoul
  beauty shopping,
    189–98
  dermatologists, 189

facials, 186–87
favorite spas, 184–85
hair salons, 187–88
nail shops, 185–86
neighborhoods, 176–80
restaurants, ordering
    at, 180–82
shopping tips, 182–84
subway and taxi,
    198–99
wifi, 200
Sephora, 201
serums, 71, 109
sheet masks, 74–79,
    109–10
Sik, Son Dae, 155, 196
skin
    acid mantle on, 40, 42
    cells, shedding, 47–48,
    52
    primary function of,
    31
    sagging, 84
skin cancer, 81, 83, 86,
    88, 96, 97–98, 166
skin-care products,
    117–33
    for age groups, 124
    cosmeceutical, 125
    dermatologist
        recommended, 124
    expiration dates, 126
    hypoallergenic, 124–25
    for men, 123–24
    mixing and matching
        brands, 127

natural, "chemical
    free," 125–26
new ingredients in,
    130–31
prices of, 123
skin types and, 117–19
Skinfood, 196
skin softener, 42
skin stories
    Dave Cho, 99
    India-Jewel Jackson,
    62–63
    Jenn Im, 202–3
    Kim Ju Won, 79
    Paul Kang, 132–33
    Son Dae Sik, 155
    Soo Joo Park, 44
    Yeon-seo Oh, 115
    Young Ah Kim, 26–27
skin types
    combination, 122
    dry, 119–20
    normal, 119
    oily or acne-prone,
    120–21
    sensitive, 122
sleep, 160–61
sleeping packs, 73–74
smoking, 165–66
snail mucin, 76
snail secretion filtrate, 131
soap, 40
sogaetings, 16–17
soju, 166
Soko Glam, 18–19, 99,
    200

Son & Park, 196
Son & Park Beauty
    Water, 155
spas. See Korean spas
spritzing, 142
steam rooms, 55
stearyl alcohol, 43
stratum corneum, 68
stress, 162
subway and taxi, 198–99
sugar scrubs, 49
Sulwhasoo, 197
Su:m37, 196
sunblock, 87
sunglasses, 94–95
sun protection. See also
    sunscreen
    myths and facts, 84–98
sunscreen, 81–99
    for acne-prone skin,
    121
    after exfoliating, 52,
    113
    chemical-based, 89
    for children, 96–97
    in daily routine, 92
    ears, neck, and
        shoulders, 98
    hands and lips, 98
    ingredients in, 86–87
    mineral-based, 88, 97
    for no-makeup look,
    152
    nongreasy, 94
    PA rating system, 91
    physical, 88